362.10942
VAN

nch
12.12.06

362.106.809
VAN

Clinical Governance in Primary Care

KT-417-198

Second Edition

Edited by

Tim van Zwanenberg

Professor of Postgraduate General Practice
University of Newcastle upon Tyne

and

Jamie Harrison

General Practitioner
Associate Director of Postgraduate GP Education
University of Newcastle upon Tyne

Foreword by

Sir Michael Rawlins

Chairman
National Institute for Clinical Excellence

Radcliffe Medical Press Ltd
18 Marcham Road
Abingdon
Oxon OX14 1AA
United Kingdom

www.radcliffe-oxford.com
The Radcliffe Medical Press electronic catalogue and online ordering facility.
Direct sales to anywhere in the world.

British Library Cataloguing in Publication Data

A catalogue record for this book is available from the British Library.

ISBN 1 85775 861 7

Typeset by Advance Typesetting Ltd, Oxfordshire
Printed and bound by TJ International Ltd, Padstow, Cornwall

Contents

Foreword

Clinical governance is about trying to ensure that NHS patients receive the highest attainable standards of clinical care. It is a philosophy that places a responsibility on health professionals to seek ever greater improvements to the individual, collective and institutional care that patients receive from the NHS.

However, the philosophy is uncomfortable. For it implicitly accepts that we do not invariably provide our patients with the quality of care they deserve – and that although we want to do our 'best' for our patients, we sometimes depart from 'best practice'. It is also implicit that clinical governance, and the commitment it demands, can never be wholly satisfied. Yet it is in the striving, asymptotically, for the goals we seek that we are most likely to achieve them. For as we get close to utopia, the goal posts will change and more will be required of us.

This second edition of *Clinical Governance in Primary Care* extends and amplifies the principles outlined in the first edition. It explains and explores clinical governance in all of its multifaceted dimensions. It will instruct and enthuse all those involved in delivering care to patients, and will bring clinical governance alive.

Sir Michael Rawlins
Chairman, National Institute for Clinical Excellence
Ruth and Lionel Jacobson Professor of Clinical Pharmacology,
University of Newcastle upon Tyne
September 2003

Preface

So what is clinical governance?

A man that looks on glass, on it may stay his eye; or if he pleaseth, through it pass, and then the heaven espy.

George Herbert

How comprehensive is our gaze? How willing are we to explore the world, and let it survey us? Even before the current power of globalisation, it had become clear to many that clinicians could no longer live in isolation, from either themselves, their colleagues or their clients (patients). The arrival of clinical governance is a public recognition of that fact.

The themes of clinical governance are those of quality, accountability, transparency and continuous improvement. It is said that such concerns can only flourish in a context of co-operation, teamwork and support. Much is made of the need to develop a 'no-blame' culture, yet ultimately someone or some group must take responsibility, and someone must lead.

In the light of such a discussion, many differing pictures of clinical governance have emerged, each with its own interest group. It is interesting to speculate on how to complete the sentence beginning 'Clinical governance is…'.

A window

The verse from George Herbert's hymn reminds us that to look upon a window offers us two choices. We can focus on the glass itself (near focus) or look beyond it (distant focus). The near focus will hold us to a near, familiar view of our world – a limited horizon, where familiarity may breed complacency.

Better to look through the window, to gain the broader horizon and the challenge of the bigger picture. With that may come a glimpse of heaven, but equally an inkling of the road that must be travelled to get there. In this sense, clinical governance is the means by which organisations begin to see what their true objectives are.

A mirror

Windows also reflect light, as mirrors on the world. Some of the components of clinical governance can act like that, feeding back information, as they do, on what we are like, how we are doing. There are those who avoid the presence of mirrors.

Mirrors are valuable tools – ask any dentist, ENT surgeon, shaver or beautician. The reflections of the mirrors within clinical governance inform the thinking of teams and practitioners in the health service. They cannot, of course, ensure that any action is taken as a result. They are merely inert commentators, companions on the journey.

A system

System development, or systemisation, would be seen, by many, as the answer to difficulties in primary care. The problem is not, they would argue, the individuals concerned, but the context in which such individuals work together.

Certainly, teaching about how to initiate and develop systems in primary care has been slow for clinicians. Better management has, however, begun to rectify this. Clinical governance allows this process to accelerate, as the need for both good management systems and care pathways is highlighted.

A culture

To bring about cultural change is always difficult. Such change must be accompanied by a clearly articulated vision of what is envisaged, be realistic and well supported – financially and with human resources – and be seen as beneficial to all stake-holders. Otherwise, the change will only be superficial and cosmetic.

Clinical governance encourages a culture of excellence, partnership and account-ability. As such, it must also find the resources to sustain its high ideals and maintain its vision across all the players in primary care.

An education

Some would wish to see clinical governance as purely an educational exercise. Clearly, the need for education about clinical governance, in addition to the clear role for continuing professional development within clinical governance itself, is self-evident.

Yet there is a danger that the educational element could take over the whole agenda. It must see itself in partnership with the drive to better systems in primary care, and in the evolution of the culture of mutuality, trust and excellence which is already present in much of primary care.

A stained glass window

Returning to George Herbert, we may wish to finish with another type of window. A stained glass window comprises many differently coloured panes of glass, each set in place to form a coherent whole. Individually, each pane may be monochrome, uninspiring. Put all the panes together and a totally different effect emerges – a story told or an image expressed.

The components of clinical governance considered individually may not add up to much. Each is rather a building block, or a coloured pane, in the construction of a larger and more significant work of art. Only when viewed in its entirety can such a work be judged. Lose one component and the story is incomplete, the image marred. Each component on its own is not enough.

Tim van Zwanenberg
Jamie Harrison
September 2003

List of contributors

Richard Baker Director, Clinical Governance Research and Development Unit, University of Leicester

Arthur Bullough Head of Primary Care Service Management, County Durham and Darlington Primary Care Support Unit

Sir Liam Donaldson Chief Medical Officer, Department of Health, London

Martin Eccles Professor of Clinical Effectiveness, University of Newcastle upon Tyne

Christina Edwards Director of Nursing, County Durham and Tees Valley Strategic Health Authority

Beverley Ellis Senior Lecturer in Health Informatics, Lancashire Postgraduate School of Medicine and Health

Ruth Etchells Theologian and formerly Vice Chair, Durham Family Health Services Authority and Chair of its Medical Services Committee

Robbie Foy Clinical Senior Lecturer in Primary Care, University of Newcastle upon Tyne

Debbie Freake General Practitioner and Medical Director, Newcastle Primary Care Trust

Allan Gillies Professor of Information Management, Lancashire Postgraduate School of Medicine and Health

Janet Grant Professor of Education in Medicine, Open University

Jeremy Grimshaw Director of the Clinical Epidemiology Programme, Ottawa Health Research Institute

Jamie Harrison General Practitioner and Associate Director of Postgraduate GP Education, University of Newcastle upon Tyne

Robert Innes Vicar of Belmont and Part-time Lecturer in Theology, University of Durham

Mayur Lakhani Lecturer, Clinical Governance Research and Development Unit, University of Leicester

Pauline Pearson Senior Lecturer, School of Medical Education Development, University of Newcastle upon Tyne

Mike Pringle Professor of General Practice, University of Nottingham

Sir Michael Rawlins Chairman, National Institute for Clinical Excellence

Marianne Rigge Director, College of Health

Stephen Rogers General Practitioner, North London and Associate Medical Director, Islington Primary Care Trust

Alice Southern Practice Manager, Collingwood Surgery, North Shields

John Spencer Professor of Medical Education in Primary Health Care, University of Newcastle upon Tyne

Will Tapsfield Executive Partner, Collingwood Surgery, North Shields

George Taylor Director of Postgraduate General Practice Education in Yorkshire and Associate Dean, University of Leeds

Richard Thomson Professor of Epidemiology and Public Health, University of Newcastle upon Tyne

Ian Watt Professor of General Practice, University of York

Tim Wilson General Practitioner, Wallingford

Linda van Zwanenberg Head of Corporate and Clinical Governance, Newcastle Primary Care Trust

Tim van Zwanenberg Professor of Postgraduate General Practice, University of Newcastle upon Tyne

About this book

Who is it for?

We hope everyone involved in primary care will find useful information in this book. Clinical governance is after all 'everybody's business'. Primarily we have aimed to meet the needs of those charged with leading the development of clinical governance at the level of primary care trust and primary care team. The contents should be of interest and relevance to all professional groups, although we recognise that much of the material is drawn from general practice and community nursing, with less reference to the other allied professions.

For simplicity we have used the term *primary care trust* throughout, recognising that this is the organisational arrangement in England. There are equivalent primary care organisations, with different names, in the other parts of the United Kingdom. The issue of clinical governance is generic to them all.

What does it contain?

The book is intended to provide a description of the principles of clinical governance in primary care, and practical information about many of its component processes. In general, definitions, evidence and practical experience have been emphasised. Many of the chapters point to other sources of information. We have made no attempt at a detailed description of the supporting structures and processes which are being developed on a national basis to support clinical governance – in England, the National Institute for Clinical Excellence, the National Clinical Assessment Authority, the Commission for Health Audit and Inspection, the National Patient Safety Agency and National Service Frameworks. Moreover, we have tried to provide information that might be useful to primary care staff in implementing, for example, national guidelines.

How to use it?

The book is divided into three parts. The first part (Chapters 1–4) sets the scene. The conceptual and political origins of clinical governance are traced, and the significance of organisational culture is emphasised. The importance of patients, healthcare staff and processes is highlighted. Examples are given of clinical governance in action in a primary care trust and a primary care team. The second part (Chapters 5–17) is arranged around four domains of clinical governance, namely humane care, clinical effectiveness, risk management, and personal and professional development. It describes a range of practical processes that support the development of clinical governance. The third part (Chapters 18–20) looks ahead, offering a critique of how professionalism might develop in the future against a background of increasing expectation.

Readers will have different interests and can use the book accordingly.

- You may wish to read the book from page 1 to the end.
- You may have a specific interest in clinical audit (Chapters 8–10) or complaints (Chapter 13).
- You may need to understand the pressure for accountability in the NHS (Chapters 1, 5 and 19).
- You may want to consider the implications for education and training (Chapters 15–17).
- You may keep hearing about 'poor performance' and want to know more (Chapters 1 and 14).

Acknowledgements

We are grateful for the support and help of a wide variety of people in producing this book. In particular, we would like to thank all the contributors for their enthusiasm and hard work. Many colleagues have helped to clarify our thinking by asking questions and making comments on presentations that we have given on the subject in various parts of the country. Stuart Warrender gave us the idea that clinical governance is like a stained glass window. Murray Lough's paper on clinical governance in primary care in Scotland stimulated us to think about the domains of clinical governance. Christina Edwards advised us on nursing matters. We thank them all for their thoughtful ideas and comments. We have, as ever, relied on our primary care team colleagues at Collingwood Surgery, North Shields, and Cheveley Park Medical Centre, Durham. They have given us not only examples of good practice, but also constant reminders of reality. We thank our wives for their support, and their forbearance at dining rooms yet again submerged beneath papers. Radcliffe Medical Press has encouraged us throughout, and Angela McLaughlin has worked with great calm and good humour to produce the final typescript. Our considerable thanks are due to them.

Clinical governance is a system through which NHS organisations are accountable for continuously improving the quality of their services and safeguarding high standards of care by creating an environment in which excellence in clinical care will flourish.

Gabriel Scally and Liam Donaldson

Clinical governance is a framework for the improvement of patient care through commitment to high standards, reflective practice, risk management, and personal and team development.

Royal College of General Practitioners

Primary care is first contact, continuous, comprehensive and co-ordinated care provided to individuals and populations undifferentiated by age, gender, disease or organ system.

Barbara Starfield

PART 1

Setting the scene

CHAPTER 1

Clinical governance:
a quality concept

Sir Liam Donaldson

If you always do what you always did, you always get what you always got.

Granny Donaldson

> This chapter defines clinical governance and describes its origins. Clinical governance involves ensuring that quality assurance, quality improvement and patient safety are part of the everyday routines and practices of every healthcare organisation and every clinical team. Recognising the importance of organisational culture to the success of clinical governance in the new primary care trusts is vital.

Introduction

Clinical governance was one of the central ideas in a range of proposals to modernise the National Health Service (NHS) contained in a White Paper produced by the incoming Labour government in the late 1990s.[1]

From the post-war years at the beginning of the NHS, through the 1960s, to the periods of cost containment in the 1970s and 1980s, and into the era of health system reform of the early 1990s, concepts and methods of quality in healthcare underwent a quiet revolution.

In the early years of the NHS, quality was implied, assured by the training, skill and professional ethos of its staff. Standards of care were undoubtedly high for their time, and the nationalisation of health services and facilities brought about by the creation of the NHS undoubtedly improved many past inequalities in access and provision. However, quality was essentially viewed through paternalistic eyes, with the patient a passive recipient of care. The 1960s saw a growth in thinking about concepts of quality, much of it emanating from North America, notably Donabedian's quality triad (structures, processes and outcomes),[2] which has endured over more than 30 years. Despite these more sophisticated notions of quality emanating from academics and health service researchers, the vision was seldom realised in practice.

By the 1980s, management was beginning to become established within the health systems of many parts of the world. In the NHS, accountability for the performance of a health organisation came as career general managers replaced health service administrators.[3] Initially resented by many professional staff, management gradually extended to the running of clinical services with the creation of clinical directorates and budgets.

The desire to build on these trends led, in the late 1980s and early 1990s, to attempts to design incentives for efficiency and quality into the NHS system itself. The resulting internal market for public healthcare in the UK split responsibility for the purchasing and provision of healthcare between health authorities and general practice fundholders (which were allocated budgets to purchase) and NHS trusts (which competed to provide services and gained a share of these budgets).[4] The theory was that the internal market would simulate the behaviour of a real market and drive up quality while reducing costs. This concept of quality improvement remained controversial, and many professional staff working within the NHS were not confident that it could or did work.

During the 1990s, a series of high-profile instances of failed care among NHS service providers caused widespread public and professional consternation and sustained media criticism. During this time, incidents and events within local health services became public in a way that would not have been conceivable in the early years of the NHS. Traditional deferential attitudes towards doctors and others in positions of authority were changing as UK society became more consumer orientated. This was reflected in the way in which the media challenged and accused health service providers that had been responsible for incidents involving poor standards of care in which patients had been harmed or had died. Many such events in the past would not have seen the light of day at all, or if they did would have been explained away in general terms and quickly forgotten.

In the media climate of the late twentieth century, patients' deaths were no longer mishaps or unfortunate accidents. They were scandals in which, although the plight of the victim was highlighted, as much emphasis was placed on identifying those perceived as responsible.

The watershed in public and professional attitudes towards serious failures in the standards of healthcare was undoubtedly the events which took place in the Bristol children's heart surgery service during the late 1980s and early 1990s. Bristol appeared to be a statistical outlier for mortality after surgery, particularly in relation to one type of operative procedure. Despite concerns within the hospital, attempts to address and resolve the problems of clinical performance were inadequate. It was left to a 'whistleblower' – an anaesthetist – to bring the matter to external attention. At one point the surgeons were asked not to proceed with a heart operation on a particular child, but they judged the risks to be acceptable and proceeded, only for the child to die post-operatively.

What led to particular outrage when these events became public through disciplinary hearings and media reports[5] was the extent to which clinical decisions were being made on behalf of parents rather than with them. A major public inquiry into the Bristol affair[6] drew attention to a 'club culture' which was detrimental to high-quality care.

This and other cases of failed care[7,8] gave the impression of an NHS culture which at times subordinated patient safety to other considerations, such as professional loyalty, an unwillingness to challenge traditional practices and a fear of media exposure. However, they did pave the way to major reform in the way in which quality and safety were managed within the NHS.

Organisations and people

The NHS underwent a major process of reform, beginning in 1998,[1] which focused on developing primary care as the organisational locus for assessing and meeting local health needs and for commissioning and funding health services for their populations.[9]

NHS reform has also placed an emphasis on modernisation – of facilities and infrastructure, of professional practice, of organisational systems and ways of working and of attitudes towards the patient as a consumer of care.

At the heart of the process of reform has been the establishment and implementation of a clear framework for quality. This has involved setting clear standards for the NHS as a whole, formulated through a variety of mechanisms, but most importantly a National Institute for Clinical Excellence (NICE)[10] and a series of National Service Frameworks covering priority areas of care (e.g. coronary heart disease and mental health).[11–13]

It has created robust mechanisms of inspection. The Commission for Health Improvement (or, from 2003, the Commission for Health Audit and Inspection) visits local NHS organisations, reviews quality and makes public reports.[14,15]

The quality framework also requires healthcare organisations to fulfil a statutory duty of quality.[16] This means implementing satisfactory 'clinical governance' arrangements. The concept of clinical governance[17,18] has been the driving force behind improvement in local NHS services. It seeks to establish in every healthcare organisation the culture, leadership, systems and infrastructure to ensure that quality assurance, quality improvement and patient safety activities are part of the everyday routines of every clinical team. A national clinical governance development team has undertaken a major programme of change management to fulfil this aim.[19,20]

Clinical governance is essentially an organisational concept. This is made clear by the way in which it was first defined, as 'a framework through which NHS organisations are accountable for continuously improving the quality of their services and safeguarding high standards of care by creating an environment in which excellence in clinical care will flourish'.[16]

The elements of accountability, of ensuring that positive outcomes are delivered and of creating the right environment for good practice to flourish are all organisational features. Organisational culture – what it constitutes, what determines whether it is beneficial and how to change it – has not on the whole been studied systematically in the healthcare field, although it features extensively in the management sciences research literature.[21] However, there are a number of generic features which many health service managers and professionals would recognise from their good and bad experiences during the progression of their careers (*see* Table 1.1). Yet achieving the right culture is seen as the most important element in implementing the clinical governance programme within the NHS.[22]

Much of the past work on improving quality through organisational development within the NHS has been directed at hospital or community health services rather than at primary care. Although a general practice, with its extended primary

Table 1.1 Ten key features of a positive culture within a health organisation

- Good leadership at all levels
- Open and participative style
- Good internal communication
- Education and research valued
- Patient and user focus
- Feedback on performance routine
- Good use of information
- Systematic learning from good practice and failure
- Strong external partnerships
- Produces leaders of other health organisations

care team, was certainly an organisation, it was small in scale; the framework of accountability was diffuse and devolved, and the element of management was firmly in support of clinical activities rather than leading and placing responsibilities on the health professionals within the practice.

The creation of 300 primary care trusts in England (*see* Figure 1.1) changed all of this.[23] Primary care trusts serve average populations of around 170 000 and contain as many as 50 general practitioners. They have boards and chief executives.

The new primary care structures are thus substantial new organisations which are creating their own cultures. Individual general practitioners and other health professionals will become committed to success at the corporate level, as well as at the level of their own clinical teams. In setting out the agenda for the new NHS, and in particular the primary care organisations, the UK government has described this as a long-term agenda for development.

Well into the twenty-first century, primary care trusts are developing as organisations, leaving behind the small-practice ethos of the early years of the NHS. This organisational development task includes building into the new organisations a working model of clinical governance.

The first stages of implementation of clinical governance involve four key steps.[22]

1 Establish leadership, accountability and working arrangements.
2 Carry out a baseline assessment of capacity and capability.
3 Formulate and agree a development plan in the light of this assessment.
4 Clarify reporting arrangements for clinical governance within board and annual reports.

One possible model (*see* Figure 1.2) would see different members of the team taking responsibility for key functions, such as ensuring that different aspects of the quality improvement programme are 'joined together', that the important information and information technology needs of the programme are being met, that an overview of progress is taken and that communication is effective.

Whatever the leadership arrangements, essential elements are that the whole organisation is involved in a way that promotes inclusivity, and that there is clear leadership and communication from the top (*see* Table 1.2).

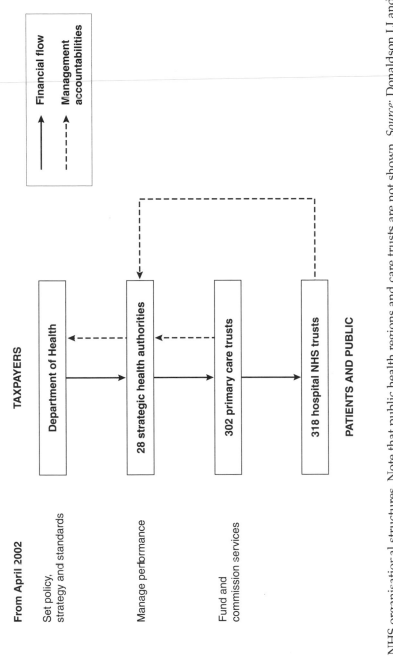

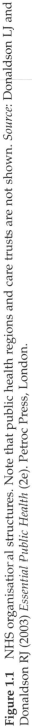

Figure 1.1   NHS organisational structures. Note that public health regions and care trusts are not shown. *Source:* Donaldson LJ and Donaldson RJ (2003) *Essential Public Health* (2e). Petroc Press, London.

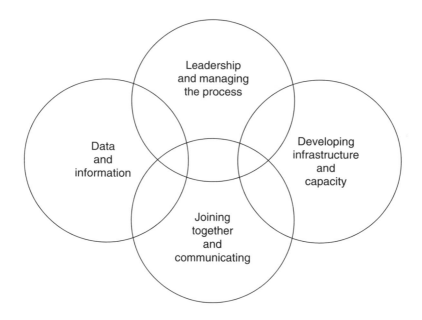

Figure 1.2 Developing clinical governance: leading change.

Table 1.2 Clinical governance: key elements of leadership arrangements

- *Inclusivity*: ensuring that all key groups in the organisation are involved and kept fully informed about the purpose and progress of the clinical governance programme.
- *Commitment from the top*: reporting and having free access to the chief executive and the board, particularly when problems need to be resolved or barriers to progress have been identified.
- *Good external relationships*: forging strong, open, working partnerships with health organisations and other agencies in the locality.
- *Constancy of purpose*: keeping the programme on course and not being deflected from the goals that the organisation has set itself.
- *Accounting for progress*: being able at all times to provide a comprehensive overview of progress with the clinical governance programme throughout the organisation.
- *Communicating*: to all staff in the organisation and to external partners on a regular basis.

A thorough analysis of the organisation's services from a quality perspective to identify their strengths and weaknesses establishes the baseline from which a development plan can be drawn up.

In closing the gap between the current position and the desired future state of improved quality, a number of questions need to be addressed (*see* Table 1.3).

Table 1.3   Closing the quality gap in a service: some important questions

- Is the solution a workforce one (more staff, different skills)?
- Is the solution an education and training one (development of existing staff)?
- Is the solution a realignment with patients' perspectives on quality (greater involvement of service users and carers in planning the improvements)?
- Is the solution an infrastructure one (new facilities or equipment)?
- Is the solution to remedy information deficits (better information, information technology, access to both)?
- Is the solution substantial investment of new resources (prioritisation through the local spending plans)?

Shifting the quality curve

A simple composite measure of quality, if one existed, would see healthcare organisations distributed along a curve (*see* Figure 1.3), with the worst performers at the left-hand tail and the leading-edge organisations at the right. The greatest impact on quality (i.e. the biggest move of the curve towards the right) will be achieved by shifting the mean – in other words, helping organisations whose performance is average (or just above or just below average) to achieve the levels of the best. However, the two tails of the distribution cannot be ignored. Poor organisational performance and serious service failure are phenomena which are probably uncommon in relation to the totality of healthcare provided in the NHS. Thus eliminating them would not cause the quality curve to shift a great deal overall. Nevertheless, such events have very serious, sometimes catastrophic repercussions for individual patients and their families. Specific incidents are often portrayed by

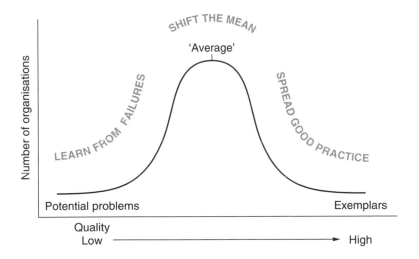

Figure 1.3   Variation in the quality of organisations. *Source*: Scally G and Donaldson LJ (1998) Clinical governance and the drive for quality improvement in the new NHS in England. *BMJ*. **317**: 61–5.

the media as if they were the tip of an iceberg of similar problems within health services. Thus their occurrence, and the media criticism which attends them, can damage public confidence in services.

Relatively little research has been conducted to explore reasons why health organisations fail. Experience suggests that organisations which are poorly led, which are defensive to criticism, which have no ethos of teamwork and where there are weak management systems will be those that are prone to failure.[18]

Finding ways to learn lessons from service failure within primary care trusts is an important part of clinical governance, and is a manifestation of their becoming effective organisations.

The activities of sharing and adopting good practice concentrate attention on the right-hand tail of the quality curve in Figure 1.3. They will help to shift the overall curve to the right, but there are other reasons for concentrating on good practice. First, it is not something which the NHS has been good at in the past. Thus patients in one part of the country will have benefited from an innovation in service delivery, while those elsewhere will have been denied its benefit. This is surely inequitable. Secondly, sharing good practice encourages a learning approach to service development and is likely to have other quality spin-offs in the type of culture that it creates. Thirdly, an increasing amount of clinical decision making will be based on following good practice guidelines, so a similar ethos needs to be developed in service organisation and delivery – recognising models of service which can be transferred to other services to create improved quality.

The emergence of the evidence-based medicine movement, which started in Canada[24] and rapidly became international in its scope, has encouraged the adoption of more rigour in clinical decision making. Numerous examples[25] exist of research evidence having been slow (or having failed entirely) to enter routine practice, so that suboptimal care is delivered to patients. The philosophy of evidence-based medicine has provided the impetus for the standards-based approach to quality.

Addressing these issues in primary care trusts is perhaps not as straightforward as it is in specialist areas of hospital medicine. This is partly because of the degree of uncertainty in many patient encounters in primary care, and the absence of a diagnostic label on which there is a strong body of research evidence with regard to clinical effectiveness. Nevertheless, promoting an evidence-based culture means ensuring that all health professionals have been trained in the critical appraisal of research evidence. It means having available and knowing how to access specialist information resources (such as that provided by the Cochrane Collaboration[26]). It also means ensuring that health professionals in primary care are able to use evidence in the interest of clinical audit and other quality-improvement methodologies.

Less experience has been gained in evaluating service models than in evaluating clinical interventions. A 'good' service (say) for diabetic people will often gain its reputation by being valued by patients and referring practitioners, rather than by formal evaluation. If the NHS is to ensure that good practice is replicated, then ways will have to be found of identifying the organisational ingredients that amount to success.

Patient safety: a key strand of clinical governance

Policy in the UK has focused on two separate dimensions of patient safety, both of which are contained within the overall clinical governance framework.

The first addresses the problem of the poorly performing practitioner. Of course, it is important to recognise that the vast majority of adverse events are not indicative of, or attributable to, deep-seated problems of poor performance on the part of individual clinicians. The causes of error are manifold and complex, and can rarely be attributed solely to the actions of one individual. Nevertheless, there are some instances where the poorly performing practitioner is at the heart of the problem. Such situations were badly dealt with by the NHS in the past.[27]

Incompetence, misconduct and ill-health-impaired performance traditionally became visible late in the day with some kind of serious incident. Too often investigation revealed a problem practitioner who had been well known in the locality for years. The issue had not been confronted, and patient safety was compromised.

In a national healthcare system it is not acceptable for a local primary care service to withdraw the practising rights of an impaired physician, leaving him or her to disappear, only to become a problem elsewhere in the country.

This aspect of patient safety has been addressed by creating a new national specialist service, the National Clinical Assessment Authority (NCAA), to which referrals of doctors with problems can be made. This service assesses the general practitioner or hospital specialist using expert advisers, and makes a recommendation for action, with an emphasis on retraining or rehabilitation where possible.[28]

The NHS now understands much more about poor practitioner performance, and has mechanisms to identify it early on, to assess it rigorously and to identify solutions. In this way patients are not exposed to unnecessary risk for long periods, and impaired performance is viewed as a problem to be fixed – not (as previously) as grounds for punishment.

For the individual practitioner it will mean keeping up to date, participating to the full in the clinical governance programme of the primary care trust, and recognising problems with his or her own performance and seeking help. Importantly, it will no longer be acceptable professional behaviour to fail to draw attention to concerns about serious problems with regard to a colleague's standard of practice.

The second dimension of patient safety, and the aspect that is now becoming very familiar to healthcare policy makers worldwide, is the risk associated with medical error occurring in unsafe systems. The whole field of medical error is becoming much more extensively researched (*see* Figure 1.4). The systems perspective is the key to understanding medical error and to improving safety.[29]

The turning point in the UK was the publication of the report *An Organisation With a Memory*.[30] This drew attention to the absence within the NHS of a reliable way of identifying serious lapses in standards of care (or medical errors), analysing them, systematically learning from them and introducing change (both locally and throughout the health service) to prevent similar events occurring again elsewhere. Drawing on research in England[31] which used similar methodologies to studies conducted in the USA[32] and Australia,[33] the report estimated that the problem in England was affecting about 10% of inpatient hospital admissions (*see* Box 1.1).

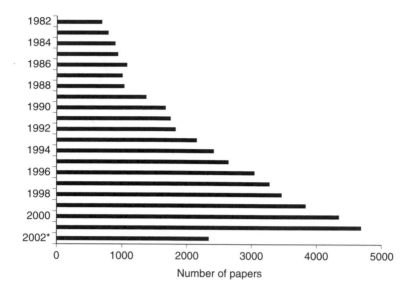

Figure 1.4 Papers in peer-reviewed journals on patient safety and medical error. *Up to end of August 2002.

Box 1.1 Size of the problem of avoidable harm in the NHS: key facets

- An estimated 850 000 adverse events in NHS hospitals per annum
- Costs of £2 billion in additional bed days alone
- Costs of £400 million per annum in clinical negligence litigation settlements
- Nearly 7000 adverse events per annum involving medical devices
- Costs to the NHS of hospital-acquired infection estimated at £1 billion a year

Source: Department of Health (2000) *An Organisation With a Memory: Report of an Expert Group on Learning From Adverse Events in the NHS*. The Stationery Office, London.

Drawing on the experience of other industries with a more embedded safety culture, *An Organisation With a Memory* called for a similar approach in the NHS (*see* Box 1.2).[30]

Serious adverse events occurring across the NHS continue to reinforce the need for action with regard to the design and safety features of medical devices and the packaging and labelling of medicines. Recent high-profile cases include the death of another 18-year-old leukaemia patient from an intrathecal injection of vincristine (a drug for intravenous use only), the death of a small child who was given nitrous oxide instead of oxygen, deaths of babies from overdoses of digoxin, potassium chloride being mistaken for sodium chloride, and lignocaine being mistaken for water.

Box 1.2   Recommendations from *An Organisation With a Memory*[30]

- A mandatory scheme for reporting adverse events and near misses in the NHS, available as a confidential service for staff to use
- Encouragement of a reporting culture in the NHS
- A unified system for analysing and disseminating lessons from adverse healthcare events and near misses
- Better use of existing sources of information on adverse events and help for staff to access the learning from previous adverse events
- Basic research into adverse healthcare events in the NHS
- Action to ensure that important lessons are implemented quickly and consistently

---

A follow-up implementation report *Building a Safer NHS for Patients*, which was published in April 2001, set out a programme for addressing the recommendations of *An Organisation With a Memory*, and established a National Patient Safety Agency.[34]

The two key elements for making health systems safer are a method for identifying and characterising adverse outcomes of healthcare actions, and the putting in place of changes that enable learning through analysis of trends and patterns of adverse events and near misses, that reduce risk and that improve patient safety. The remit of the National Patient Safety Agency extends to ensuring that adverse event reporting also takes place in primary care.

Fundamental to reporting and surfacing safety problems is the development of a culture in healthcare that is open and fair, and in which risks are assessed and patient safety has a high priority. There is a circular and consequential relationship between the development of an open and fair culture and improving safety for patients.

The proposed extension of the powers of the General Medical Council (GMC) to determine every five years whether a doctor is fit to continue in practice (so-called revalidation),[35] and the broadened concept of the duties of a doctor as set out by the GMC,[36] will also serve to increase the protection of patients and promote high standards of practice in primary medical care.

Conclusions

Undertaking clinical governance involves learning from experience of both good and bad practice. It involves addressing the diverse aspects of quality improvement which are carried out to some extent in all organisations, but also ensuring that they are performed well and systematically everywhere, and that this is achieved within an integrated quality strategy.

Clinical governance is a powerful and comprehensive mechanism for ensuring that high standards of clinical care and patient safety are maintained throughout the NHS, and that the quality of services is continuously improved. Primary care services are at the centre of a programme to modernise the NHS contained in a ten-year plan for investment and reform set out by the UK Government in 2000.[37]

Primary care organisations are developing a clinical governance culture with all that this entails for their constituent practices and practitioners. This means a commitment to corporate goals and strategies, the creation of leadership and accountability arrangements, and above all the establishment of the right ways of working at all levels. Clinical governance must be woven into the fabric of all primary care organisations. In the long term the prize to be gained is enormous, as the benefit of improved quality flows to patients up and down the UK.

Practical points

- Initiatives aimed at improving quality in the past have not been integrated.
- Clinical governance is a mechanism to ensure that quality assurance, quality improvement and patient safety are part of everyday routines and practices.
- Achieving the right organisational culture in primary care organisations will be critical to success.
- Learning from adverse events in primary care will enable risk to be reduced and patient safety to be enhanced.
- Learning from and reproducing good practice are also crucial.
- Many of the problems of poor professional practice should be prevented by clinical governance.
- Clinical governance must be 'woven into the fabric' of every primary care organisation.

References

1   Department of Health (1997) *The New NHS: modern, dependable*. The Stationery Office, London.
2   Donabedian A (1966) Evaluating the quality of medical care. *Milbank Memori Fund Q.* **4**: 166–206.
3   Griffiths R (1983) *NHS Management Enquiry*. Department of Health and Social Security, London.
4   Department of Health (1989) *Working for Patients*. The Stationery Office, London.
5   Smith R (1998) Regulation of doctors and the Bristol inquiry. Both need to be credible to both the public and doctors. *BMJ.* **317**: 1539–40.
6   Kennedy I (2001) *Learning from Bristol: the report of the public inquiry into children's heart surgery at the Bristol Royal Infirmary 1984–1995*. The Stationery Office, London.
7   Dyer C (1998) Obstetrician accused of committing a series of surgical blunders. *BMJ.* **317**: 767.
8   Redfern M (2001) *The Report of the Royal Liverpool Children's Inquiry*. The Stationery Office, London.
9   Department of Health (2001) *Shifting the Balance of Power Within the NHS: securing delivery*. Department of Health, London.
10 NHS Executive (1999) *Faster Access to Modern Treatment: how NICE appraisal will work*. NHS Executive, Leeds; www.doh.gov.uk/nice/appraise.htm

11   Department of Health (2000) *National Service Framework for Coronary Heart Disease.* Department of Health, London.
12   Department of Health (1999) *National Service Framework for Mental Health: modern standards and service models for mental health.* Department of Health, London.
13   Department of Health (1998) *National Service Frameworks.* Department of Health, London.
14   Commission for Health Improvement (2000) *Investigation into Carmarthenshire NHS Trust: report to the Assembly Minister for Health and Social Services for the National Assembly for Wales.* Commission for Health Improvement, London.
15   Commission for Health Improvement (2002) *Clinical Governance Review: the Hillingdon Hospital NHS Trust.* The Stationery Office, London.
16   Department of Health (1998) *A First-Class Service: quality in the new NHS.* Department of Health, London.
17   Scally G and Donaldson LJ (1998) Clinical governance and the drive for quality improvement in the new NHS in England. *BMJ.* **317**: 61–5.
18   Donaldson LJ and Gray JAM (1988) Clinical governance: a quality duty for health organisations. *Qual Health Care.* **7 (Supplement 1)**: S37–44.
19   Halligan A and Donaldson LJ (2001) Implementing clinical governance: turning vision into reality. *BMJ.* **322**: 1413–17.
20   Halligan A (1999) How the National Clinical Governance Support Team plans to support the development of clinical governance in the workplace. *J Clin Govern.* **7**: 155–7.
21   Ferlie EB and Shortell S (2001) Improving the quality of health care in the UK and USA – a framework for change. *Milbank Q.* **79**: 281–316.
22   Department of Health (1999) *Clinical Governance: quality in the new NHS.* Department of Health, London.
23   Department of Health (2002) *Shifting the Balance of Power: the next steps.* Department of Health, London.
24   Evidence-based Medicine Working Group (1992) Evidence-based medicine: a new approach to teaching the practice of medicine. *JAMA.* **268**: 2420–5.
25   Donaldson LJ (1996) Impact of management on outcomes. In: M Peckham and R Smith (eds) *Scientific Basis of Health Services.* BMJ Books, London.
26   Cochrane Library (1998) *The Cochrane Collaboration.* Issue 5. Update Software, Oxford.
27   Donaldson LJ (1994) Doctors with problems in an NHS workforce. *BMJ.* **308**: 1277–82.
28   Department of Health (1999) *Supporting Doctors, Protecting Patients.* Department of Health, London.
29   Reason J (1990) *Human Error.* Cambridge University Press, Cambridge.
30   Department of Health (2000) *An Organisation With a Memory: report of an Expert Group on Learning From Adverse Events in the NHS.* The Stationery Office, London.
31   Vincent C, Neale G and Woloshynowych M (2001) Adverse events in British hospitals: preliminary retrospective record review. *BMJ.* **322**: 517–19.
32   Brennan TA, Leape LL and Laird NM (1991) Incidence of adverse events and negligence in hospitalised patients. *NEJM.* **324**: 370–6.
33   Wilson RM, Runciman WB, Gibberd RW, Harrison BT and Hamilton JD (1995) The Quality in Australian Health Care Study. *Med J Aust.* **163**: 458–71.
34   Department of Health (2001) *Building a Safer NHS for Patients: implementing 'An Organisation With a Memory'.* Department of Health, London; www.doh.gov.uk/buildsafenhs

35 Irvine D (1999) The performance of doctors: the new professionalism. *Lancet*. **353**: 1174–7.
36 General Medical Council (1995) *Good Medical Practice*. General Medical Council, London.
37 Department of Health (2000) *The NHS Plan: a plan for investment, a plan for reform*. Department of Health, London.

CHAPTER 2

Clinical governance in primary care

Tim van Zwanenberg and Christina Edwards

The good of the people is the chief law.

Cicero

This chapter describes how clinical governance involves a coherent range of activities, which together assure the quality of clinical care. The involvement of patients, the support and development of staff, and proper attention to processes are important aspects of clinical governance. Accreditation and inspection by external agencies provide validation of an organisation's internal governance arrangements.

In recent years, primary care has moved to take up an increasingly pivotal position in the NHS, such that the relatively newly formed primary care trusts in England (and their equivalent primary care organisations in the other countries of the UK) are responsible not only for managing primary care, but also for commissioning much of secondary care, and for improving public health. Against this background of increased power, influence and responsibility, accountability for the quality of primary care has inevitably assumed greater importance. Primary care trusts are now responsible for the clinical governance of primary care – giving patients, healthcare professionals, managers and government assurances about the goodness of clinical care provided.

The pressure for this level of accountability arose, in part, from the public interest in the celebrated cases of malpractice. However, even amidst the furore after the Bristol case, cautionary voices sounded. Richard Smith, editor of the *British Medical Journal*, observed that if the case led 'to an environment where we concentrate on removing bad apples rather than on improving the whole system, then both patients and doctors will suffer'.[1] Professor David Hunter pointed out that 'dependence on trust in the medical profession may not be fashionable in an age of consumerism, but that does not lessen its validity'.[2] Both were commenting specifically on doctors, but the same principles apply to all healthcare professionals. Mechanisms are needed which help to develop all, and which rebuild trust.[3]

There are three further reasons for the heightened interest in the quality assurance of primary care. First, there are evident differences in the range of services provided, and there is significant variation in the quality of those services. And although there have been improvements in some aspects of the quality of care, achieved at modest cost during a time when the NHS was undergoing a series of reforms, significant improvements are still possible. A longitudinal study of 23 practices in England compared quality of care in 2001 with that delivered in 1998. Organisational access to services, the organisation of chronic disease management and the quality of angina care all improved, but there were no significant changes in the quality scores for mental healthcare, elderly care, access or interpersonal care. Furthermore, considerable variation remained among the practices studied.[4]

Secondly, these inconsistencies have never been fully remedied by the many attempts at quality improvement in the past. Too often initiatives have been taken up only by the 'leading-edge' primary care teams. And in general, programmes of development have had only one component (e.g. the development of clinical audit) and have been isolated from one another. This has resulted in fragmentation[5] and a good deal of frustration among progressive primary care professionals and managers. That said, the broader approaches to quality improvement which have characterised recent programmes are not without their disadvantages. Few research data are available to show whether they work or are cost-effective. However, equally there is no conclusive evidence that there are no benefits or that resources are wasted.[6] The problem is that such quality programmes, like clinical governance, are large-scale complex interventions applied to equally complex organisations in a changing context with many short- and long-term outcomes, few of which can be unambiguously attributed to the intervention, at least with current research methods. For the time being it may be more sensible to concentrate on identifying critical success factors, as judged by different parties, and on refining measurable primary care quality indicators. Undoubtedly the greatest weakness of the clinical audit programme has been the failure to 'close the loop' (i.e. to change practice or services in the light of audit findings).

This leads on to the third factor behind this modern focus on quality, which is the development of valid and reliable quality indicators for primary care. Most quality indicators are used in hospital practice, but much work has been carried out over the last few years to define quality and its parameters in primary care and then to refine indicators of it. In particular, the National Primary Care Research and Development Centre has developed a useful conceptual framework for quality, which it suggests can be defined as a combination of three parameters – access to care, clinical effectiveness and interpersonal effectiveness.[7]

Clinical governance in primary care

Thus clinical governance offers a coherent framework for bringing together the disparate strands of quality improvement. The original government White Paper, *The New NHS: modern, dependable*, identified ten component processes of clinical governance, and proposed that a 'quality organisation' will ensure they are in place.[8] Each of these processes is the subject of a chapter in this book. They have been called 'the ten commandments of clinical governance', but in truth there could have been only eight or nine (a number of components overlap) or 11 or more (some important components were not listed). Indeed, two more (chapters) have been added to the original ten for the second edition of this book. They concern information management and teamwork (*see* Box 2.1).

Box 2.1   The '10 (now 12) commandments of clinical governance'

1 Evidence-based practice with the infrastructure to support it (*see* Chapter 6)
2 Good practice, ideas and innovations systematically disseminated (*see* Chapter 7)
3 Quality improvement processes (e.g. clinical audit) (*see* Chapter 8)
4 High-quality data to monitor clinical care (*see* Chapter 9)
5 Effective management of information (*see* Chapter 10)
6 Clinical risk reduction programmes (*see* Chapter 11)
7 Adverse events detected and openly investigated – and the lessons learned promptly applied (*see* Chapter 12)
8 Lessons for clinical practice systematically learned from complaints made by patients (*see* Chapter 13)
9 Problems of poor clinical performance recognised at an early stage and dealt with (*see* Chapter 14)
10 All professional development programmes reflect principles of clinical governance (*see* Chapter 15)
11 Leadership skill development at clinical team level (*see* Chapter 16)
12 Effective teamworking (*see* Chapter 17)

The significant point is that each on its own will not suffice. The processes, some of which are quite narrow whereas others are more broad, need to be linked so that clinical governance becomes 'a systematic set of mechanisms'[9] or 'a systematic joining up of initiatives to improve quality',[10] which provides primary care organisations with the right balance of accountability and continuous improvement. Most of the activities involved in clinical governance were happening already, more or less – some more, some less. The main idea is to promote and marshal all of the activities to develop the organisation as a whole.

The outcome of an early workshop on clinical governance that involved patient representatives, primary care practitioners and health service managers is pertinent here. The participants concluded that the arrangements for clinical governance in primary care would have to meet a number of paramount needs:

• the need to secure public confidence – including the involvement of patients and carers from the start
• the need to be inclusive of all practitioners
• the need to support the continuous improvement of the many (who are trying to do their best)
• the need to map and make use of existing resources
• the need to provide an explicit and effective process for dealing with unacceptable practice.

At each level of primary care – individual, practice, primary care team and primary care trust – success will depend on the interaction of the three key parts of the system, namely patients, people (i.e. staff) and processes (*see* Box 2.2). For example, it is well known that compliance with advice is dependent on the relationship between doctor and patient.

Box 2.2   The three key contributors to clinical governance in primary care

Patients
- They want to contribute and hold the NHS in high regard.
- They should be involved early on.
- The purpose of their involvement should be clear.
- Evidence-based practice is of little use if patients do not follow it.
- They can help to ensure that performance measures are realistic.

People
- They make primary care work – it is a 'people business'.
- They need to be valued and supported.
- They must demonstrate continuing fitness to practise.

Processes – internal
- The '12 commandments of clinical governance'.
- They need to be systematically joined up.

Processes – external
- Professional re-licensure.
- Support (e.g. National Clinical Governance Support Team).
- Accreditation (e.g. Improving Working Lives).
- Inspection (e.g. Commission for Health Audit and Inspection).

Patients

Although there has been much rhetoric about the involvement of patients, not only in decisions about their own care but also in planning service development and in enhancing the quality of care, and there are plenty of examples of good practice, effective involvement is by no means universal. Much of the early experience, in general practice at least, was focused on studies of patient satisfaction, yet responding to a questionnaire hardly constitutes engagement. Practice-based patient participation groups have been tried, and in some cases provide at least a useful vehicle for two-way communication. However, they are perceived by many as being the preserve at best of the middle classes, and at worst of special interest groups or lobbies.

Yet the argument for involvement is irrefutable. There is a need to 'move to an active rather than passive trust between doctors and patients, where doctors share uncertainty'.[1] For so long as the health service sustains a paternalistic attitude, patients will respond like children and not help with negotiating the inevitable trade-offs in everyday practice. Primary care is a public service that responds very largely to public demand. In an age of consumerism and arguably of suspicion, practitioners in primary care have had to adjust to new demands for responsiveness, accessibility, quality and service. The debate now is not so much *whether* patients should be involved, but *how*. As with other aspects of clinical governance (e.g. risk reduction), there is much to learn from the techniques employed by commercial service industries. They steadfastly avoid tokenism, learn constantly from customer feedback (especially complaints), and use a range of proactive methods for giving and receiving information (e.g. focus groups, customer panels, and so on).

Ruth Chambers' book, *Involving Patients and the Public: how to do it better*, provides a useful starting point on the dos and don'ts of patient involvement, and she has some important advice:

> You have to be sincere about wanting to involve patients and the public in making decisions about their own care or about local health services for any such exercise to be successful. You cannot expect ordinary people to put forward their views or take part in any discussion if they think that decisions have already been made and the consultation is just a public relations exercise.[11]

In particular, the purpose of the patient involvement needs to be clear, and the most effective methods for incorporating patients' views need to be used. The methods used to determine patients' views can be divided into three types, namely measures of preferences, evaluations of users, and reports of healthcare. The type of measure used will depend on what aspect of healthcare is being assessed (*see* Box 2.3).[12]

Box 2.3   Preferences, evaluations and reports

Preferences
- These are ideas about what should occur in healthcare systems.
- They are often used to refer to individual patients' views about their clinical treatment.
- The term 'priorities' is used to describe the preferences of a population.

Evaluations
- These are patients' reactions to their experience of healthcare (i.e. whether the process was good or bad).

Reports
- These are objective observations by patients on the organisation or process of care.
- They are made regardless of patients' preferences or evaluations. For example, patients can note how long they had to wait for an appointment, irrespective of whether this was too long or not.

Source: Wensing and Elwyn[12]

People

Primary care is a 'people business', and the quality of care provided depends critically on adequate numbers of caring, competent and motivated staff, and the ability of those staff to work as a team. There is a danger that, in an effort to ensure practice is safe and effective, complex and time-consuming monitoring systems will be developed, rather than the focus being on developing the people, their clinical practice and teamworking. The current vogue for performance management as the main managerial technique deployed in the NHS means that clinical leaders have to be especially alert to avoid this trap.

There are important technical aspects of 'human resource management' which go beyond the scope of this book. Nevertheless, primary care organisations – both trusts and practices – are having to get to grips with such matters as workforce planning, occupational health and the proper procedures for recruitment, selection, induction, appraisal and discipline of staff. For example, in one of the most notorious untoward incidents in nursing in recent years (the Amanda Jenkinson case), much hinged on the accuracy of references in support of job applications and who had the authority and training to write them.[13] Indeed, these responsibilities with regard to employment are becoming more challenging as primary care organisations:

- seek to recruit doctors and nurses from overseas – they require considerable pastoral support, language training and adequate induction
- campaign to persuade practitioners who have left the service to return, often after several years' absence – they need career counselling, assessment of their educational needs and individually tailored retraining
- strive to retain staff and delay early retirement
- implement annual appraisal for all – the important educational needs that are identified have to be met
- take on healthcare services in prisons – many of the staff require top-up training, and have been unused to providing clinical supervision for less experienced colleagues
- develop local procedures for tackling practitioners whose performance is a cause for concern – they require careful and professional assessment and remedial education
- take on increasing responsibility for the scrutiny and support of GP non-principals registered on their Supplementary Medical List.

Of particular significance in the context of clinical governance is the issue of personal stress and its effects on the workforce and patient care. Interest in stress has developed apace as organisations have recognised that it costs them vast amounts of money – through absence and litigation, and the fact that unhappy, tense, tired or anxious practitioners do not produce quality care. Stress and all of its related problems arise both in the workplace and in the individual. Individual causes may stem from personality or background, whereas job-related factors include lack of sleep, poor communication and poor teamwork. It is known that better teams have less stressed staff, probably because they support each other, notice when one person is performing below par, and step in to help.[14] Therefore, in the pursuit of clinical governance, primary care organisations would do well to support and value their staff and invest in the development of effective teams (*see* Chapter 17).

The continuing personal and professional development of staff (*see* Chapter 15) and the development of leadership (*see* Chapter 16) are covered elsewhere, but there are three related areas which merit discussion here, namely scope of professional practice, appraisal and clinical supervision, and professional re-licensure.

Scope of professional practice

Over the last two decades general practitioners have taken on new roles, both in clinical care (e.g. minor surgery, care of patients with diabetes, and recently even more specialised areas such as urology clinics) and in the corporate management of the health service through their involvement in primary care trusts. They have done so without recourse to a higher authority, and have in the past expressed frustration at their nursing colleagues' apparent inability to do the same at their behest!

This situation has changed as nurses have also extended their roles and some have become nurse practitioners. In 1992, the then regulatory body for nurses, the United Kingdom Central Council for Nursing and Midwifery (UKCC) (since replaced by the new Nursing and Midwifery Council), published *The Scope of Professional Practice*.[15] This replaced the 'extended role of the nurse' provision whereby doctors delegated tasks to nurses and had to certify the nurse's competence. The aim was to allow nurses to undertake new and expanding roles while continuing to safeguard patient safety. The document asserted that 'each nurse is accountable for their own practice and that it is their professional judgement which can provide innovative solutions to meeting the needs of patients and clients in a health service that is constantly changing'.

The Scope of Professional Practice was withdrawn on 31 March 2002 when the Nursing and Midwifery Council came into being. The Code of Professional Conduct was issued on 1 April 2002 and came into effect on 1 June 2002. The Code, which describes accountability and safety in nursing and midwifery practice, incorporates the elements of the pioneering document *The Scope of Professional Practice*.

Thus any nurse can take on responsibilities outside their traditional role provided that they adhere to the following principles. Nurses taking on new roles must:

- be satisfied that patient needs are uppermost
- aim to keep up to date and develop personal skills and competence
- recognise the limits to their personal knowledge and skill, and remedy any deficiencies
- ensure that existing nursing care is not compromised by taking on new developments and responsibilities
- acknowledge personal accountability
- avoid inappropriate delegation.

This approach has allowed much greater flexibility and creativity in the development of nursing practice in response to patient needs, without nurses having to collect endless certificates. However, it does place the onus on the practitioner to define the limits of their competence within the overall *Code of Professional Conduct*, and the clinical governance of the care provided relies heavily on the proper development of any extension of nurses' roles.

This has relevance for doctors and other professionals in primary care who are seeking to change or develop their range of skills. The appointment of general practitioners with special clinical interests (GPWSIs) is an important element of health service policy in the UK. Some may be 'accredited' by gaining a diploma or the equivalent, but all will need to adhere to the principles outlined above, particularly with the advent of revalidation. Through revalidation doctors will have to demonstrate that they are fit to practise in *all* aspects of their professional work. It has further been proposed that primary care organisations will need a framework for addressing the quality and standards issues raised by the development of new services, which depend on GPWSIs. This would enable the doctors to be properly accredited.[16]

Appraisal and clinical supervision

Clinical supervision is normal professional practice for a number of the 'caring' professions (e.g. counsellors, psychotherapists), and was well established in midwifery long before clinical governance came into being, and before most other professions had formalised the process. It has been defined as follows:

> a formal process of professional support and learning which enables individual practitioners to develop knowledge and competence, assume responsibility for their own practice, and enhance consumer protection and safety in complex clinical situations.[17]

In essence it involves protected time for the practitioner(s), either individually or in a group, with a supervisor. The time is used in a structured way to reflect on practice, to review critical incidents and to identify means of personal and practice development. Despite being endorsed by the UKCC in 1996,[18] the development of clinical supervision in nursing has remained patchy, with disciplines such as midwifery and psychiatric nursing leading the way. However, the concept of supervision has gained acceptance with the widespread introduction of the process of appraisal across the NHS, which has been defined as follows:

> a positive process to give someone feedback on their performance, to chart their continuing progress, and to identify development needs. It is a forward-looking process essential for the developmental and educational planning needs of the individual.[19]

Annual appraisal is now mandatory for all general practitioners, and the effective implementation of appraisal for all staff is a key part of clinical governance for primary care organisations, and the main vehicle for planning individuals' and organisations' programmes of continuing professional development (*see* Chapter 15). Appraisal for general practitioners is also intimately linked with their revalidation, which in turn leads to their re-licensure.

Professional re-licensure

The Government sees professional self-regulation as one of three major elements contributing to the quality assurance of NHS healthcare, the others being clinical governance and lifelong learning.[20] Whereas clinical governance might be said to apply to services, which are provided collectively by organisations or teams, professional self-regulation is concerned with the fitness of individuals to practise. The Government and others have argued successfully that effective clinical governance needs enhanced professional regulation, and important changes are under way.

The newly formed Nursing and Midwifery Council and the Health Professions Council (the regulatory body for healthcare professionals other than doctors and nurses) both have reformed structure and functions that:

- give them wider powers to deal effectively with individuals who pose unacceptable risks to patients
- create smaller Councils
- streamline the professional registers
- provide 'explicit powers to link registration with evidence of continuing professional development'.[21,22]

Thus the former UKCC's Professional Registration and Practice (PREP) requirements, which were introduced in 1995,[23] will be built on. These formalised for the first time the requirement for continuing professional development. Under this each nurse must undertake a minimum of five days of study every three years, and must also maintain a personal profile detailing their professional development.

The process is of relevance to doctors as the General Medical Council introduces revalidation. In May 2001, the Council confirmed that in the future and for the first time all doctors would have to demonstrate on a regular and periodic basis that they remained fit to practise in their chosen field. This process was termed revalidation, and through revalidation doctors would be entitled to remain registered with the Council and thereby remain licensed to practise. The introduction of revalidation was said to represent a significant change in the traditional approach to medical regulation, which until the 1990s had remained largely unchanged since 1858, when the Council was first established.[24]

Now all doctors are being issued with licences to practise, and these will be renewed every five years on satisfactory completion of the process of revalidation. Most general practitioners will be able to achieve revalidation by confirming that they have taken part in a managed annual appraisal system based on the General Medical Council's *Good Medical Practice*. This places an onus on primary care organisations to ensure that the quality of their system of appraisal is properly assured.[25]

Processes

Clinical governance depends on the deployment of a coherent range of processes internal to the organisation or team, many of which are described in the following chapters. There are three external processes which apply to the organisation, in contrast to professional re-licensure of the individual. These are support, accreditation and inspection.

Support

The NHS Clinical Governance Support Team was established in 1999 to support the development and implementation of clinical governance. The team is now part of the Modernisation Agency. Its aims are to promote the goals of clinical governance throughout the health service, to act as a focus of expertise, advice and information, and to offer a training and development programme for clinical teams and NHS organisations.[10] It also supports trusts rated as 'nil star' by the Commission for Health Improvement to deliver an action plan through its Rapid Response Unit, which was formed in 2002.

The team runs a clinical governance development programme for multidisciplinary delegate teams drawn from organisations across the NHS. Delegate teams attend a series of five task-oriented workshops (learning days) punctuated by eight-week action intervals spread over a period of nine months. During this time delegates lead project teams as they review, design and deliver quality improvement initiatives.

Primary care trusts can obtain similar support for focused service development and organisational development from other sections in the Modernisation Agency (e.g. the Primary Care Collaborative and the National Primary Care Trust Development Team, NatPact).

Accreditation

There has been a growing interest in accreditation as a form of composite measure of quality assurance for primary care organisations. Accreditation has been defined as 'a system of external peer review for determining compliance with a set of standards'.[26]

It involves review of an organisation's performance by external agents. Performance is measured against a set of agreed criteria and explicit standards, and a report of the results is provided to the organisation. Accreditation can be used for a variety of purposes, but the examples in primary care are mainly focused on quality improvement (*see* Box 2.4).

Box 2.4 Accreditation programmes in primary care

Training practices	Joint Committee on Postgraduate Training in General Practice (JCPTGP)
Membership by assessment of performance (MAP)	Royal College of General Practitioners
Fellowship by assessment (FBA)	Royal College of General Practitioners
Quality Practice Award (QPA)	Royal College of General Practitioners
Quality Team Development (QTD)	Royal College of General Practitioners

Accredited Professional Development (APD)	Royal College of General Practitioners
Primary care research team assessment (PCRTA)	Royal College of General Practitioners
ISO 9000 (formerly BS 5750)	British Standards Institute
Investors in People	Learning and Skills Councils
Improving Working Lives	Strategic Health Authorities
European Business Excellence Award	European Framework for Quality Management
Health Quality Service Award	King's Fund (formerly known as Organisational Audit)

In their evaluation of accreditation in primary care, Walsh and Walshe[27] suggested a number of questions that primary care organisations should ask before embarking on any particular scheme.

1 Is the primary purpose quality improvement, and how clear are the objectives?
2 Is participation voluntary, and how many organisations have taken part in the past?
3 At what level are the standards set, and how were they developed? What do they cover, and how are they measured?
4 Which data are required for assessment, and what methods are used? Who are the external assessors, and how were they selected and trained?
5 How is the feedback to be provided, and is it confidential to the organisation?
6 What is known of the impact on or benefit to organisations that participate, and what are the follow-up arrangements?
7 What fees are charged and (most importantly) what are the opportunity costs in terms of time and preparation?

A programme of accreditation for the primary care teams in a primary care trust could prove a useful mechanism for the development of clinical governance. It would certainly offer the possibility of a consistent external review across teams.

Inspection

The Commission for Health Improvement (CHI) was established following the publication of the 1997 White Paper, *The New NHS: modern, dependable*.[8] Its key functions were defined as follows:

- clinical governance review – routine, rigorous assessment of every NHS organisation
- investigation – (usually at the behest of the Secretary of State) to investigate systems when things have gone seriously wrong

- national studies – studies of the implementation of National Service Frameworks and National Institute for Clinical Excellence guidelines
- leadership – disseminating good practice.[28]

To date, CHI has taken a wholly developmental approach to its routine inspections of clinical governance arrangements, and has been prepared to change and modify in its visits and reports in the light of experience and feedback.[29] That said, its scoring system contributes to the star rating of hospital trusts, and primary care trusts and mental healthcare trusts are to be similarly star rated from 2004.

CHI is now being succeeded by the Commission for Healthcare Audit and Inspection (CHAI), with much enhanced responsibilities. It has incorporated the Office for Information on Healthcare Performance, and is thus managing the national patient and NHS staff surveys. This is consistent with CHI's original aims of keeping their reviews patient centred and focused on staff development. CHAI is also set to manage the national clinical audits and organisational performance assessment, including an improved star-rating system.

CHAI will inspect every part of the NHS and private healthcare, will review the quality of patient care and how well the NHS is using its funds, and will produce an annual report to Parliament on the state of the NHS. It is independent of the NHS and Government. Its functions will cover all of CHI's original functions, the National Care Standards Commission's responsibilities for inspecting the private health sector, and the Audit Commission's value-for-money studies in health.

Primary care trusts can now anticipate an inspection by CHAI on a regular four-year cycle. It remains to be seen whether this 'super-inspectorate' will improve patient care or simply add to the burgeoning bureaucracy.[3,29]

Conclusion

Two questions are commonly asked by primary care staff. What is clinical governance and what is their role in it? The first two chapters should have gone some way towards answering the first of these questions. The answer to the second question depends to some extent on the role of the individual. The chief executive of the primary care trust has overall responsibility as the 'accountable officer' for both corporate and clinical governance in their organisation. The clinical governance lead for a primary care team or trust will oversee and direct the many processes that contribute to clinical governance, but they cannot do it all themselves, nor can they do it all at once. This is a programme of development that will take place over a period of some years.

The individual practitioner is responsible for demonstrating their continuing fitness to practise, as well as for contributing to the collective quality assurance of the service provided to patients – clinical governance.

Practical points

- There is pressure for greater accountability for the quality of primary care.
- Unacceptable variations in quality still exist.
- There has been fragmentation of the many past initiatives aimed at quality improvement.
- Clinical governance provides a coherent framework for the systematic linking of activities.
- Patients and carers need to be involved.
- Primary care staff need to be valued and supported through mechanisms such as appraisal and clinical supervision.
- All practitioners will have to demonstrate their continuing fitness to practise on a periodic and regular basis.
- Collective clinical governance depends on the deployment of a range of internal processes.
- These can be enhanced through external support, accreditation and inspection.

References

1   Smith R (1998) All changed. Changed utterly. *BMJ*. **316**: 1917–18.
2   Hunter D (1998) A case of under-management. *Health Serv J*. **25 June**: 18–19.
3   Harrison J, Innes R and van Zwanenberg T (2003) *Rebuilding Trust in Healthcare*. Radcliffe Medical Press, Oxford.
4   Campbell S, Steiner A, Robison J *et al*. (2003) Is the quality of care in general medical practice improving? Results of a longitudinal observational study. *Br J Gen Pract*. **53**: 298–304.
5   Thomson R (1998) Quality to the fore in health policy – at last. *BMJ*. **317**: 95–6.
6   Øvretveit J and Gustafson D (2003) Using research to inform quality programmes. *BMJ*. **326**: 759–61.
7   Campbell S, Roland M and Buetow S (2000) Defining quality of care. *Soc Sci Med*. **51**: 1611–25.
8   Department of Health (1997) *The New NHS: modern, dependable*. The Stationery Office, London.
9   Department of Health (1999) *Clinical Governance: quality in the new NHS*. Department of Health, London.
10 Halligan A and Donaldson L (2001) Implementing clinical governance: turning vision into reality. *BMJ*. **322**: 1413–17.
11 Chambers R (2000) *Involving Patients and the Public: how to do it better*. Radcliffe Medical Press, Oxford.
12 Wensing M and Elwyn G (2003) Methods for incorporating patients' views in health care. *BMJ*. **326**: 877–9.
13 North Nottingham Health Authority (1997) *Report of the Independent Inquiry Into the Major Employment and Ethical Issues Arising From the Events Leading to the Trial of Amanda Jenkinson (the Bullock Report)*. North Nottingham Health Authority, Bassetlaw.

14 Firth-Cozens J (2001) Interventions to improve physicians' well-being and patient care. *Soc Sci Med*. **52**: 215–22.

15 UKCC (1992) *The Scope of Professional Practice*. UKCC, London.

16 Gerada C and Limber C (2003) General practitioners with special interests: implications for clinical governance. *Qual Prim Care*. **11**: 47–52.

17 Department of Health (1993) *A Vision for the Future*. Department of Health, London.

18 UKCC (1996) *Position Statement on Clinical Supervision for Nursing and Health Visiting*. UKCC, London.

19 Department of Health (1999) *Supporting Doctors, Protecting Patients*. Department of Health, London.

20 Department of Health (1998) *A First-Class Service: quality in the new NHS*. The Stationery Office, London.

21 Department of Health (2001) *Establishing the New Nursing and Midwifery Council*. Department of Health, London.

22 Department of Health (2001) *Establishing the New Health Professions Council*. Department of Health, London.

23 UKCC (1997) *PREP and You*. UKCC, London.

24 General Medical Council (2000) *Changing Times. Changing Culture*. General Medical Council, London.

25 General Medical Council (2003) *A Licence to Practise and Revalidation*. General Medical Council, London.

26 Scrivens E (1995) *Accreditation: protecting the professional or the consumer?* Open University Press, Buckingham.

27 Walsh N and Walshe K (1998) *Accreditation in Primary Care*. Health Services Management Centre, University of Birmingham, Birmingham.

28 Patterson L (2001) Commission for Health Improvement (CHI). *J Med Defence Union*. **17**: 14–15.

29 Wilson T (2002) What's in an acronym? *J Clin Govern*. **10**: 111–12.

CHAPTER 3

Clinical governance in action – in a primary care trust

Linda van Zwanenberg and Debbie Freake

Therefore, the Trust might be expected to be a particularly apt form of organisation for the delivery of healthcare, with qualities that would not be expected, for example, in a profit-making public limited company.

Robert Innes[1]

Primary care trusts (PCTs) are relatively new organisations at varying stages of development. This chapter describes how one large city PCT has developed its approach to clinical governance.

Introduction

Primary care groups (PCGs) and their successor primary care trusts (PCTs) were one of the key changes heralded in the government White Paper, *The New NHS: modern, dependable.*[2] They were to provide the framework in primary care for the NHS to discharge its new statutory duty of quality.[3] Each PCG (and later PCT) needed to ensure that a set of interlinked processes was in place which together would provide the right balance of public accountability and continuous quality improvement of clinical services.[4]

Primary care groups (operating as subcommittees of the then health authorities) made significant progress in developing the infrastructure to support clinical governance. However, the evolution to trusts from October 2001 onward brought new responsibilities for assuring the quality of commissioned hospital services, for providing community health services and for improving the health of the population. More recently, the PCTs have taken on even more of the responsibilities previously borne by health authorities, particularly with regard to the other primary care contractor professions – the dentists, the optometrists and the pharmacists.[5]

The implementation of clinical governance at the level of a PCT is different to implementation at the level of a practice or clinical service, and poses different challenges. The PCT is a public authority incorporating clinicians who are both directly employed staff and independent contractors. Inevitably the organisation is more at arm's length from direct patient care, and it needs to ensure that arrangements for the governance of all of its 'business', including clinical care, are sound. This is a complex task, but in broad terms (and for the sake of simplicity) it involves three main interdependent areas of endeavour:

1 promoting good practice in clinical governance among practices and clinical services – providing leadership and facilitation
2 controls assurance – an NHS audit system of corporate governance arrangements which involves self-assessment by trusts against NHS-wide minimum standards in three domains, namely governance, financial management and risk management
3 clinical negligence scheme for trusts (CNST) – an NHS collective insurance scheme, which includes an audit system for assessing the management and mitigation of clinical risks.

Developments in governance

Corporate governance in both private and public sector organisations has assumed greater importance during the past decade, in the light of a series of high-profile corporate failures (e.g. Barings Bank and Enron). The principles by which organisations are managed and the effectiveness of the systems that they have in place to meet their objectives and to identify and manage risk have increasingly been scrutinised. The NHS has adopted many of the requirements that have been promoted or imposed in the private sector. For example, all companies listed on the London Stock Exchange are required to maintain a system of internal control (controls assurance) by conducting a thorough and regular evaluation of risks. They are also required to report to shareholders on an annual basis that they have done so by publishing a Statement of Internal Control (SIC).

Boards of all NHS organisations are now also required to provide a similar annual assurance that there are robust systems in place across the organisation to meet objectives and to manage risks to those objectives. The rationale behind this is that effective governance and risk management increase the probability of success and reduce the possibility of failure and the uncertainty of achieving the organisation's overall aims. A consistent conclusion of public inquiries into cases of organisational failure and serious untoward incidents is that poor systems are often to blame, rather than necessarily the conduct of individuals.

It is not appropriate to describe in detail the NHS controls assurance system or the clinical negligence scheme for trusts in this book, but more information can be found from the Department of Health Controls Assurance website at www.doh.gov.uk/riskman.htm.

In the rest of this chapter we shall outline our approach to promoting clinical governance among practices and clinical services.

Experience in Newcastle upon Tyne

Newcastle Primary Care Trust was established on 1 April 2001. As with other PCTs, it brought together a number of organisations (*see* Box 3.1), each with its own arrangements for clinical governance, and each with a different culture and ways of working. Harmonising the approach to clinical governance across these disparate organisations has proved both challenging and rewarding.

Box 3.1   Newcastle Primary Care Trust

- Previous health authority functions and staff
- Three primary care groups – 43 GP practices
- Community nursing services from two community trusts, including health visitors, district nurses and allied health professionals
- Specialist services, including diabetes care, genito-urinary medicine, occupational health, podiatry, physiotherapy, contraception and sexual health, community dental services, health psychology, and interpreting service
- 63 dental practices
- 63 community pharmacies
- 36 optometrists

All of the above serve a resident population of approximately 280 000 people.

The three PCGs, which pre-dated the PCT, had worked well in implementing clinical governance at a locality level. The general practitioners and other clinical staff met regularly, and had built up the trust and rapport necessary for sharing information about individual practices. Such trusting relationships are crucial if there are concerns that performance is not as it should be. Keeping a 'locality focus' has therefore been an important issue in developing clinical governance further in the PCT. In particular, the majority of former fundholding practices were clustered in one locality, and they were keen to build on their innovations.

The newly formed PCT had to undertake four key steps to develop clinical governance:

1 establish leadership, accountability and working arrangements
2 carry out a baseline assessment
3 formulate and agree a development plan in the light of the baseline assessment
4 clarify reporting arrangements for clinical governance with the trust board.

Promoting clinical governance
The clinical governance strategy

The construction of a clinical governance strategy for the PCT has been critical in setting the direction of travel, in bringing together the predecessor organisations, and in gaining ownership to move forward. The strategy was developed under the auspices of the trust's Clinical Governance Committee, a subgroup of the Professional Executive Committee (PEC). The committee is chaired by a non-executive director and meets monthly. Over time it has changed its focus from being largely a business meeting to encouraging more debate about issues of strategic substance. Following the publication of *Shifting the Balance of Power*,[5] the committee was expanded to include representatives from the other contractor professions.

The process of developing the strategy included widespread consultation with PCT staff (including trade-union representatives) and patients, including Community Action on Health (a local community development network) and the Community Health Council. A baseline assessment of clinical governance activity and preparedness was initiated following the establishment of the PCT in April 2001. Arguably it was this process that ensured greater ownership and helped to make clinical governance 'everyone's business'.

The following key principles were agreed to underpin the strategy and the promotion of a quality framework.

- It meets the needs of the population that it serves.
- It recognises our staff as our greatest asset and values their skills and experience.
- It minimises risks to patients and staff.
- It secures commitment to achieving and spreading best possible clinical practice.
- It is open and accountable to local people and to the health authority.
- It promotes a supportive environment of lifelong learning.

The resultant strategy had four main strands (*see* Box 3.2). The fifth strand, namely excellence, was added not only to complete the obvious and easily memorable mnemonic, but also to encourage and recognise best practice. The strategy was ratified by the PCT board in January 2002.

Box 3.2   The clinical governance strategy

S   Staff
M   Managing and using information
I   Involving partners
L   Lifelong learning
E   Excellence

Staff

This section of the strategy covers all staff who are directly employed by the PCT and all those working in primary care settings (i.e. the contractor professions and their employed staff). This strand includes the following components.

- *Professional development and training* – developing staff with the right skills and competencies to meet patients' needs and to deliver *The NHS Plan*.[6]
- *Clinical supervision* – initially undertaking a survey of current activity; ensuring that the principles of reflective practice are promulgated within independent clinical practice.
- *Clinical leadership* – widening access to leadership development opportunities (e.g. for clinical nurse leaders); development of the Head of Service role in specialist services; leadership development for PEC members and locality groups.

- *Supporting staff* – developing the culture and infrastructure necessary to enable an appropriately supported workforce, including policies for dignity at work, protection of whistleblowers, diversity, zero tolerance of unacceptable behaviours, and flexible working; developing mechanisms to aid GPs and practice-employed staff, such as mentoring, an occupational health service, and support for GPs and staff with difficulties.
- *Professional performance* – identifying problems at the earliest possible stage in order to protect both staff and patients; development of robust appraisal and personal development planning.
- *Disciplinary action and investigation* – developing new disciplinary policies and procedures.

Managing and using information

The Clinical Governance Committee recognised that information needs to be managed in order to maximise its potential (*see* Chapter 10). It also needs to be accurate, useful and easily accessible, and the interests of patients need to be safeguarded. This strand includes the following components:

- *Information technology* – ensuring that all staff are linked to email and the Internet; making networking of community centres a priority; encouraging services to display relevant information (e.g. waiting times) on the PCT website.
- *Records management* – meeting the requirements for the controls assurance standard.
- *Patient confidentiality* – carrying out an audit of Caldicott Guardian[7] arrangements.
- *Internal communications* – encouraging electronic communications; building on existing communication channels and developing others; staff newsletters, staff forums and other staff meetings.
- *External communications* – developing an external communications strategy; addressing the needs of minority ethnic groups and those with learning or literacy difficulties; establishing communication channels with other organisations; implementing Department of Health guidance on consent for examination or treatment.
- *Audit programme* – developing a programme of audit to complement other clinical governance activity; encouraging audit as an integral part of general practice development plans.

Involving partners

It is not just clinicians and managers who need to be involved in order to make clinical governance effective. Patients and carers as well as other organisations also need to participate. This strand includes the following components.

- *Public involvement and user/patient/carer participation* – building on previous community development approaches; sharing examples of good practice; meeting targets set by the PCT's public involvement strategy group chaired by the non-executive director ('champion for public involvement').
- *Partnership working* – working with trade-union organisations and the local professional representative committees; participating in the local strategic partnership with local authority services and other bodies.
- *Tackling inequalities* –tackling inequalities in partnership with statutory, private-sector and voluntary organisations and local people; developing a strategy

for health improvement and specific strategies to include 'hard-to-reach' groups.
- *Commissioning* – ensuring that providers of commissioned and contracted services consider key quality issues; ensuring that service level agreements include agreed quality criteria.

Lifelong learning

Lifelong learning embraces a range of activities which encourage non-stop learning – learning from error, learning from research and research evidence, and learning from each other. This strand includes the following components.

- *Risk management* – implementing both clinical and non-clinical risk management; ensuring that controls assurance standards are met, particularly in relation to health and safety; handling complaints and serious untoward incidents; reviewing the complaints procedure; developing adverse event and near-miss monitoring; building on clinical risk assessment and risk management training.
- *Clinical effectiveness* – developing professionals' skills in critical appraisal; implementing National Institute for Clinical Excellence and other evidence-based policies.
- *Research and development* – developing a research-conscious workforce; implementing a research governance framework.
- *Disseminating best practice* – encouraging best practice through good practice events, displays and workshops; seeking opportunities to share good practice and learning with other organisations.

Yearly action plans have been developed from the strategy, and progress has been reported on a quarterly basis to the Clinical Governance Committee and then to the PEC and the PCT board. The clinical governance development plan, derived from the strategy, has been placed on the staff Extranet, with the relevant evidence of achievement against each objective. The strategy, together with minutes from every Clinical Governance Committee meeting, is placed on the trust's website to provide a measure of public accountability.

Clinical governance infrastructure

Newcastle is unusual among PCTs in that corporate and clinical governance have been combined, with one person appointed to head up both. This has been an important move in acknowledging the inherent tension between business management and clinical practice, while endeavouring to make sure that issues are not 'compartmentalised'. The idea is that clinical governance and the learning that goes with it should be embedded in all aspects of the organisation. The PEC ensures that clinical governance issues are kept at the forefront through regular reports to the PCT board, and the board regards clinical governance as an integral part of the corporate agenda.

In addition to a small central clinical governance support team, each locality has a GP lead for clinical governance and a part-time clinical governance manager to work at a locality level. This is intended to facilitate a 'bottom-up' approach, with ownership by front-line staff. Issues that are important to particular localities can be addressed locally. More generic issues (e.g. patients' access to services) are addressed across all localities.

Conclusion

Other PCTs will have faced the similar task of bringing different organisations and staff groups together, and managing the tension between encouraging development from below and responding to the demands for accountability from above. The value of co-ordinating all of the activities that make up clinical governance is accepted, but the complexity of it is daunting. Reflecting on clinical governance in action since the creation of the PCT brings to mind the following examples of things that have worked well:

- combining clinical and corporate governance
- 'time-out' sessions in the localities with 'back-fill' provided – this increased the attendance by GPs and practice staff
- promoting the Royal College of General Practitioners (RCGP) Quality Team Development as a vehicle for developing clinical governance at the level of the practice team
- innovative approaches to training (e.g. using actors to enhance training in handling complaints)
- good practice educational events
- establishing a professional advisory forum to foster two-way communication and to bring an additional professional perspective to clinical governance activity
- establishing a specific group to examine complaints and incidents in detail – summarised reports are submitted to the PCT board, and common themes are identified for targeted action
- an inclusive approach to the development of the clinical governance strategy
- building good relationships with trade-union representatives, and their early involvement in developing policies (e.g. the policy for the protection of whistle-blowers)
- working with internal auditors to achieve controls assurance standards.

Progress has not always been smooth, and the inevitable cavalcade of policies and strategies that comes with the establishment of any new organisation has generated a formidable programme of work. In retrospect, a framework and timetable for reviewing policies and strategies would have been helpful, in particular identifying key staff with protected time for implementation. Strategy is important as it provides purpose and direction, but it is no substitute for action.

The following outstanding matters still need to be addressed:

- discharging the PCT's public health function – the PCT has a responsibility for the safety and quality of the services it commissions and subcontracts, as well as those it provides directly to local communities
- implementing Section 11 of the Health and Social Care Act – which places a duty on NHS organisations to involve health service users at all stages
- ensuring that all staff have an awareness of risk management and are able to identify risks within their own area of work
- providing adequate training and protected time for individuals and teams.

Practical points

- PCTs are new organisations.
- They have a statutory duty to provide quality in primary care, which is discharged through a range of corporate and clinical governance processes.
- Constructing a strategy for clinical governance provides a sense of direction and an opportunity to gain ownership among clinicians.
- Developing staff, managing information, involving partners and promoting lifelong learning and excellence are all important aspects.
- Providing adequate training and protected time for individuals and teams remains a major challenge.

References

1 Innes R (2003) Macfarlane on trust and Trusts. In: J Harrison, R Innes and T van Zwanenberg (eds) *Rebuilding Trust in Healthcare*. Radcliffe Medical Press, Oxford.
2 Department of Health (1997) *The New NHS: modern, dependable*. The Stationery Office, London.
3 Department of Health (1999) *Clinical Governance: quality in the new NHS*. Department of Health, London.
4 Baker R, Lakhani M, Fraser R and Cheater F (1999) A model for clinical governance in primary care groups. *BMJ*. **318**: 779–83.
5 Department of Health (2001) *Shifting the Balance of Power Within the NHS: securing delivery*. Department of Health, London.
6 Department of Health (2000) *The NHS Plan: a plan for investment, a plan for reform*. Department of Health, London.
7 Department of Health (1999) *Caldicott Guardians*. Department of Health, London.

CHAPTER 4

Clinical governance in action – in a practice

Will Tapsfield and Alice Southern

Where GPs have worked in a wider team, established baseline information about their work as it really is, set agreed targets for improved
work by the whole team, and then repeated the cycle of audit and innovation at a pace the team can accept as reasonable, care of high blood
pressure, type 2 diabetes, and chronic lung disorders are as good as in
any hospital clinic, and better in that patients with multiple problems
(that is, most patients) can be dealt with by people they know, close to
their homes.

Tudor Hart J (1988) *A New Kind of Doctor*. Merlin Press, London

This chapter describes some of the features of clinical governance as implemented by a busy urban practice in the north of England. In common with
many others, the practice has grown in size and complexity and in the range
of services provided. A range of quality assurance mechanisms is used.

Introduction

For most people most of the time, the functional unit of primary care in the UK is
the primary care team based on a general practice in all its myriad variety. Effective clinical governance must therefore be implemented at this level. Historically,
the variation in size and organisation of practices, together with a lack of clear
information about what they do, has made it difficult to establish any sensible
system of accountability for quality at an individual practice level. And despite
many changes, the 1948 definition of GPs' work in the NHS has altered little: 'To
render to their patients all necessary and appropriate medical services of the type
usually provided by general practitioners.'[1] In other words, GPs do what GPs do
– defining their work and their own standards. The extent to which this will
change with the new GP contract remains to be seen.

Nonetheless, the challenge now is to demonstrate to patients, government and
NHS organisations and primary care team members themselves that standards are
satisfactory and are being achieved. This practice-based approach has to complement

what can be achieved by the primary care trust (PCT) (e.g. by using practice-specific performance data). Clinical governance should ensure quality care at the practice level. That is what makes the difference to patients' experiences.

The practice characteristics

Like all practices, ours is unique, and to help the reader to understand the clinical governance arrangements, some background information is given on the changes in the practice over the last 20 years (*see* Table 4.1). The practice has changed from a small business that largely ran itself into a large organisation that is actively managed and which is now well used to coping with rapid change and development. The practice moved into spacious (at the time) purpose-built premises in 1994, yet it now faces exactly the same problem as it did 20 years ago – lack of space, which is limiting development.

Table 4.1 Practice changes over a 20-year period

	1983	*2003*
Number of patients	8700	12 000
Accommodation	1 site 3 consulting rooms No offices	2 sites with IT links 11 consulting rooms 6 offices

Staff
  Doctors
  District nurses
  Health visitors
  Practice nurses
  Administrative staff
	5 (*c.* 4 wte)
	1
	1
	0
	7 (4 wte)
		9 (7 wte)
		4
		3
		3
		17 (13.5 wte)

Office equipment	1 typewriter 3 phone lines 6 phone extensions	35 personal computers 8 phone lines 35 phone extensions 4 scanning machines
Teaching and training	0	Training practice Undergraduate teaching Nursing students
External weekly sessions done by GPs	0	2 research 2 appraisal 3 mental health 1 sexual health

wte, whole-time equivalent.

Clinical governance framework

Although the practice would be hard-pressed to describe its mission, aims or management structure in formal terms, the ethos in the practice is one of offering a good service to the patients and local community, as well being supportive of and caring towards all the staff who work in the practice. The executive partner has a strong leadership role, supported by the practice manager, and both are active in the leadership of clinical governance.

In the year 2000 the practice devoted a time-out session to defining the role of the executive partner. The aim was to answer the following questions.

1 What are individuals' roles in the team?
2 What are the functions of the executive partner?
3 Are there alternative management structures?
4 If the executive partner structure continues, who is best placed to fulfil the role now *and* in the future?
5 How should the role/functions change?
6 Who should carry out what functions?
7 What are each individual's development needs:
   • to maximise team effectiveness?
   • to promote succession planning?

During the time-out session, the practice confirmed that the existing executive partner structure would continue. More importantly, the role of the executive partner was explicitly defined (*see* Box 4.1), and it included overall responsibility for clinical governance.

Box 4.1   The role of the executive partner

The executive partner has a defined leadership role, mandated by the practice. The functions of the executive partner are as follows:

• to carry overall responsibility for clinical governance
• to consider the strategic aims of the practice
• to ensure effective team functioning
• to prevent individual stress and burnout
• to balance the workload of individual doctors within and outside the practice
• to take an overview of patient relationships
• to be responsible for partnership and practice finances
• to act as the focal point for external relationships
• to match offered consultations to demand.

Baseline assessment

Before we move on to describe some of the activities that underpin clinical governance in the practice, and the specific example of the practice programme for patients with diabetes, it is relevant to present the rapid appraisal undertaken in 2001 (*see* Table 4.2) under the then so-called 'Ten Commandments' of clinical governance (*see* Chapter 2). The changes that have taken place since are shown in the second column of Table 4.2.

Table 4.2 Baseline assessment

Process	*Activity in 2001*	*Activity in 2003*
Evidence-based practice	• Some team members use the Internet • Two doctors appraise guidelines • Guideline folder in preparation • PRODIGY installed	• All team members have desktop access to the Internet and use it to access clinical information • One doctor has responsibility for appraising guidelines and deciding what goes into the practice folder • Guidelines are also available 'electronically' on the network
Disseminating good practice	• Team members occasionally circulate information from journals, courses • Regular programme of continuing professional development (CPD)	• Extensive use is made of internal email system to disseminate clinical 'titbits' • Regular journal club meetings • Experience of copying letters to patients shared through publication, and through membership of NHS Plan Copying Letters Implementation Group • Experience of in-house peer appraisal now being shared with local practices wishing to implement the process
Quality improvement processes	• Audits are undertaken fairly regularly	• Awarded RCGP Quality Practice Award • Regular audit activity continues • Mental health structured care developed following in-house training • Participation in primary care collaborative project focusing on access and ischaemic heart disease • Introduction of telephone surgeries • Move to longer consultation times – doctors can choose optimum length for their style (between 10 and 15 minutes) • Drug formulary updated

continued

Table 4.2   Continued

Process	Activity in 2001	Activity in 2003
		• Implemented recall systems for chronic disease monitoring • Extension of diabetes programme to other chronic diseases • Multidisciplinary communication skills training piloted and now part of continuing professional development programme. This includes administrative staff
Appropriate use of data	• Annual activity analysis • Audit of chronic disease management • Analysis of prescribing	• Practice has moved to being 'paper-light', so patient data are available to all clinical team members from the desktop without the need for access to notes • Developing effective working relationship with practice pharmacist, who has taken over the management of all patients who need regular drug monitoring
Reducing clinical risk	• Acknowledged lack of knowledge, activity and expertise	• Dedicated administrative support to control daily, weekly and monthly prescriptions for the elderly, vulnerable and those who abuse prescribed medication • Dedicated clinic to monitor patients on methadone • Fostering a climate within the whole team of acknowledging and learning from error at all levels • Use of computer-based 'patient notes' to provide audit trail for messages that were previously handwritten or sent by email
Significant event analysis	• Occasional formal significant event analysis meeting • Supportive team encourages 'debriefing' after near misses, etc.	• Regular learning event meetings to which all team members are encouraged to bring examples of clinical or administrative errors (*see* Table 4.3) • Occasional significant event meetings involving relatives of the patient and colleagues from secondary care

continued

Table 4.2 Continued

Process	Activity in 2001	Activity in 2003
Lessons from complaints	• Only one written complaint in the last two years • Lessons from complaints *not* shared • Not yet a culture which welcomes complaints, although informal feedback between team members is good • Exploration of patient involvement in progress	• Significant increase in the number of complaints • Multidisciplinary meetings held to discuss individual complaints and the lessons to be learned from them • Practice systems altered as a result of reflection and significant event analysis (e.g. alert messages on screen for patients with dementia)
Poor performance tackled	• Feedback among team members is the norm	• Audit of surgery waiting times for patients – excessive waiting times for some patients have led to lengthening appointment times for some doctors • An audit of cervical smear quality revealed that some doctors were not doing enough to maintain their skills – smear taking is now the responsibility of specific doctors and nurses • Cardiopulmonary resuscitation (CPR) update training for the whole team
Continuing professional development (CPD)	• Programme of weekly lunch-time multidisciplinary CPD meetings • Programme of receptionist training • Doctors have engaged in peer appraisal – with planned follow-up • Attached staff are beginning to develop personal development plans (PDPs)	• Ongoing programme of weekly clinical meetings – topics have reflected the learning and development needs defined during the appraisal process • Patient and 360-degree colleague feedback questionnaires have been introduced, and the outcome is shared and discussed • Ongoing receptionist training • Practice is a pilot site for practice-based GP appraisal as one route to fulfil Department of Health requirements

continued

Table 4.2 Continued

Process	Activity in 2001	Activity in 2003
Leadership development	• Roles of executive partner and practice manager are well established and effective • Role of nursing representative at weekly management meetings is established • Team has a good sense of direction from previous 'time-outs' set out in practice development plan	• Time-out session to identify and agree the key roles of the executive partner and to define other leadership areas in the practice (*see* above) • Exploration of re-structuring of nursing team to promote leadership

Clinical governance in action

In essence there are two questions that need to be answered.

• How do we know that the practice is providing a good service?
• How do we demonstrate to others that the practice is providing a good service?

As responsible professional people we seek a positive answer to the first question. We want to satisfy ourselves. However, we accept that we also have an obligation to our patients and our paymasters to answer the second question, and have therefore attempted to find ways of gathering internal and external feedback in a structured and objective manner.

Climate and culture

The practice positively encourages an open climate within the team so that everyone can suggest improvements in service development. The practice is open to the opinions of outsiders to the practice – whether they are professional colleagues, patients or others with a more formal role, such as the Community Health Council. This type of climate or culture is encouraged and made more effective by a variety of activities.

• *Significant event reviews*. Along the lines described in Chapter 12, these are held regularly and include all involved staff. Colleagues from outside the practice who are involved in the patient's care are also invited. This has included local consultants, nurses and the matron of a local nursing home. The deceased patient's relatives were involved on one occasion, which proved to be a particularly powerful method of learning about how others look at the quality of care. The practice has also developed what are called *learning event meetings*, at which team members are invited to present more minor incidents as vehicles for learning as a practice. The summary of such meetings is disseminated to all members of the team (*see* Table 4.3).

- *Creation of a 'dream practice'*. A time-out session for the entire practice involved everyone in 'visioning' the perfect practice to meet their own wants and needs as patients – a dream practice unlimited by the normal constraints.
- *Review of shared care services*. Local specialists are encouraged to attend annual service review and audit meetings in the practice, and are invited to give feedback on the quality of services offered by the practice.
- *Clinical educational meetings*. These regularly involve local experts in a shared discussion about the most effective way of developing a practice service.
- *Visits by members of the Community Health Council*. These visits have been encouraged to review the care offered and suggest possible improvements.
- A variety of *patient satisfaction surveys* have been tried in the practice over the years, but have generally been disappointing in terms of the information that they provide. The most recent survey, namely the Client-Focused Evaluations Programme (*see* http://latis.ex.ac.uk/cfep), which examined the standard of individual doctors' interpersonal skills, has been the most informative. However, although the results were reassuring with regard to the quality of interpersonal skills in general as well as the individual performance of the doctors, the survey has not provided much information about the best way to improve and develop the service further.
- *Contacting patients on discharge from hospital*. Practice reception staff routinely phone patients immediately on discharge to check that they are all right and have everything they require, and to ascertain whether they need advice from a doctor or nurse.
- *Copying referral letters to patients*. This began as a small, practice-based research project well in advance of *The NHS Plan*, which promised that all clinical correspondence would be copied to patients as a right.[2] The findings demonstrated to the practice how highly patients value receiving a copy of their GP referral letter.[3] The process has since been implemented as routine practice policy.

Table 4.3 Learning events meeting: summary

Case	*Learning points*
Middle-aged man being investigated by practice for cough, admitted with possible myocardial infarction, and later found to have lung cancer	• Practice responsibility to be proactive in following up investigations for potentially serious illness • Do not make any assumptions about a comprehensive or holistic assessment of patients in hospital • Beware of 'care pathways' – they do not cater adequately for wider problems
Non-English-speaking refugees not accessing essential preventive care for children	• Contact named person at PCT (named health visitor) • Language line may provide more appropriate help than interpreters • What about giving immunisation when hepatitis B status is unknown? (named doctor to research)

continued

Table 4.3 Continued

Case	Learning points
Granulation tissue due to failure to remove suture following resection of basal-cell carcinoma	• All patient transactions in the surgery must be recorded on the computer (practice manager to implement for Friday afternoon district nurse clinic) • Do not make any assumptions about hospital communications (even if it is not our responsibility)
Visiting demented patient in absence of family member with or without family conflict	• Contact Alzheimer Society for advice about technical and legal status of 'next of kin' and 'consent'; also seek advice about presence of family members in cases of suspected elder abuse (named doctor to research) • Review what is recorded and how on 'patient alerts' on computer (executive partner and practice manager)
Groin pain ultimately being identified as seriously diseased hip joint	• Beware the infrequent attender with unusual symptoms • Beware false reassurance of normal or near-normal investigation results or consultant opinion when symptoms persist
Pregnancy on progesterone-only pill (POP)	• Beware amenorrhoea in patients on the pill • Ask 'When was your last period and was it normal?', rather than 'Is there any chance you might be pregnant?' • Need teaching session on indications and relative risks/benefits of combined oral contraceptive (COC) vs. POP with regard to risks of heart disease vs. pregnancy, etc. (named doctor to action)
Appropriate investigation and/or management of shortness of breath	• Need more information on indications for (and blood bottles to be used for) D-dimers, and meaning of results (named doctor to research) • Need to explore the use of pleuritic chest pain as a 'tracker' condition (named doctor to explore)
Non-specific abdominal symptoms culminating in bowel obstruction from carcinoma (and death postoperatively)	• Remember the 'Rule of Three' (previous significant event audit meeting – date given); consider referral for any patient who is being seen for the third time for the same problem where the diagnosis is uncertain
Management of severe sore throat (i.e. pre-quinsy)	• What is the appropriate antibiotic for severe sore throat; is it clindamycin – and at what dose? (named doctor to research)

Service development

As can be seen from Table 4.1, the practice has undergone immense change, as have many others. It is a constant challenge to make sure that the practice can cope with these developments while at the same time handling the normal and continuing pressure of the ordinary workload, and maintaining the morale of the team. However, the practice recognises that innovation and service development are good for both patient care and team morale, if they are properly managed. Some recent examples of significant service development are listed below.

- Taking over a practice vacancy. A local, vacant, single-handed practice has been established as a branch surgery, using modern communication links and shared professional development to develop standards to match those of the main practice.
- Employing a nurse practitioner to complement the existing nursing team and to extend the range of services offered by nurses, including the triage of minor illnesses.
- Developing the practice as one that is 'paper-light'. About 40 people enter data into the practice clinical system, with over 500 entries per day on patients' clinical records.

The practice has found that the successful implementation of such major developments is critically dependent on good leadership and a range of processes designed to involve the team (*see* Box 4.2).

Box 4.2   Implementing service developments

- Ongoing discussion with all team members to gain full support and co-operation
- Sharing experiences at clinical meetings (e.g. copying of referral letters)
- Reviewing problems and refining systems as necessary
- Listening to feedback from team
- Ongoing training and development
- Appropriate use of skill mix within the practice across administrative and professional staff
- Consistency in approach to the use of practice systems
- Continual review and improvement of systems

Professional development

Peer appraisal

The planned introduction of appraisal and revalidation for GPs appears to have focused on the individual doctor in isolation. However, we believe that this is better achieved within a team setting. For several years now we have held group peer appraisal for the doctors in the practice, which allows the production of both personal professional development plans and a collective professional development plan linked to the needs of the practice.[4] The latter plan is used to determine much of the content of the multidisciplinary educational programme for the practice.

360-degree feedback
In 2003, the doctors in the practice participated in a structured 360-degree feedback process (Doctor Insight 360°; www.edgecumbe.com). This involved each doctor completing a self-assessment questionnaire and inviting 12 colleagues across all disciplines, including administrative staff, to complete similar questionnaires about him or her anonymously. All questionnaires were returned to the external consultants, and each doctor was provided with a compilation of the feedback comparing self-assessment with the assessment of colleagues. The feedback covered four domains of behaviour:

1 overall performance
2 clinical performance
3 performance as a professional colleague
4 performance in education and research.

The results were shared between pairs of doctors at the subsequent peer appraisal session. As with the patient satisfaction survey (*see* above), the results were reassuring – even affirming – for the individual doctors, but it was difficult to identify concrete personal development needs.

Prolonged study leave
Three partners have taken advantage of the opportunity for prolonged study leave. This has not only benefited them as individuals, but has also benefited the practice in the following ways:

1 development of a systematic approach to the provision of mental healthcare, including:
   • a structured review programme for patients with enduring mental illness
   • extension of the role and hours of the practice counsellor to enable them to tackle a wider range of mental health problems
   • introduction of the regular use by all team members of self-help literature for patients with common mental health problems
2 development as a research practice
3 development of a programme of multiprofessional communication skills training. Good communication skills are the foundation of the work that we do, yet it is rare for primary care professionals to receive training in communication skills after qualification. An ongoing programme has been developed involving the review of consultations on video or audio tape in small groups.

Formal external evaluation
We received the Royal College of General Practitioners Quality Practice Award in February 2000. Preparation for the award was a great stimulus for the team, and winning the award was a tremendous morale booster. The substantial paperwork

involved has been used extensively subsequently to continue the process of development. The assessors who visited on behalf of the Royal College commented as follows:

> The practice was 'buzzing' with energy and creation of ideas, and because of that, members of the team felt able to suggest improvements to patient care and systems. As a result, impressive innovations have occurred.

This reinforced our belief that a culture and climate of innovation is one of the key elements of effective clinical governance. We accept that there is also a need for the generation of data and reports for external checking, but the inevitable bureaucracy that this requires must not stifle the energy and enthusiasm that are needed to develop the service to improve the care of patients.

The practice programme for patients with diabetes

Finally, we shall describe the example of the practice programme for patients with diabetes, not so much for the detail of the service, but more to highlight the lessons we have learned about developing a quality service.

In 1985, the practice provided only reactive care to control the symptoms of the 87 patients who were known to have diabetes. Now, however, an organised structured programme involving considerable multidisciplinary input provides reactive and preventative care for 320 patients to a standard that is audited annually.

Arguably the programme has been successful for the following reasons:

- an enthusiastic local consultant has championed the cause of providing good care integrated between primary and secondary care
- the early and continuing involvement of a local GP in the service monitoring group
- regular multidisciplinary educational meetings held for GPs, practice nurses, diabetes specialists, chiropodists, dietitians and others
- the development of a good relationship between hospital and practices, which has developed into mutual trust.

At the start of the programme a 'leap of faith' was required, as the evidence was not as strong then. However, there is now a substantial evidential basis for the shared protocols of management. The district-wide programme now provides the following:

- a folder of protocols, guidelines and standards shared by both primary and secondary care, thus ensuring that evidence-based care is delivered across the district
- regular review of new evidence and developments undertaken by the diabetes service, discussed at educational meetings and disseminated by newsletter

- annual audit data shared between all practices and compared with secondary care data; this ensures that all practices aspire to the same standards and it highlights areas where the scheme can make improvements
- audit data collected centrally from computer records which are completed as part of routine patient care
- research data relating to the programme to inform the evidence basis for diabetes care[5]
- continuing professional development for all those involved in the care of patients with diabetes.

The practice holds an annual review-of-service meeting with colleagues from secondary care, informed by the comparative district audit data. These meetings have enabled the practice to focus on the following practice-specific issues.

- Initially all annual patient reviews were conducted at the diabetes centre at the local district general hospital. The practice now undertakes all care at a practice level for the majority of patients.
- The practice doctors and nurses involved have developed skills in looking after patients on insulin.
- There has been reorganisation of the way in which the care is provided. Due to the increase in the number of patients, much of the care is now provided outside the weekly multidisciplinary clinic.
- A dedicated administrative support worker runs the call and recall system. This has ensured the smooth running of the clinic and reduced the number of non-attenders.
- A specialist clinic has been arranged for poorly controlled type 2 patients, enabling joint review by the practice team and a local consultant and specialist nurse. This has been much more valuable as an educational exercise than simply referring the patients to the hospital clinic, and it has given the practice team greater confidence with regard to managing more complex cases.

Box 4.3 lists the elements of clinical governance that have supported the development of the practice diabetes programme. The practice has also developed programmes of care for other conditions (e.g. a shared care programme for heroin addicts, and a comprehensive programme for the prevention and management of vascular disease), and the same characteristics apply to these.

Box 4.3 Characteristics of successful programmes of care

- The whole team 'on board' and 'signed up' to the concept
- Leadership
  - in the practice – a practice champion
  - outside the practice – a consultant champion
- External relationships and support
- Staff training and ongoing education and professional development
- Accurate register
- 'Programme folder' to include evidence base, protocols and guidelines

- Protected time (i.e. a dedicated clinic)
- New resources (e.g. in-house chiropody and dietetic service for patients with diabetes, a community psychiatric nurse for drug addiction)
- Ongoing review, including regular audit
  - by peers
  - by an external expert

Practical points

- Clinical governance needs to be implemented at the level of the individual primary care team. That is what makes a difference to patients.
- The leadership role of the executive partner has been explicitly defined, and includes overall responsibility for clinical governance.
- An open climate and culture seem to be crucial, where learning and professional development are valued.
- Innovation and service development are good for patients and for team morale, but need to be actively managed.
- Shared care programmes need champions in both primary and secondary care.

References

1 Department of Health (1986) *NHS Act 1977 Regulations.* HMSO, London.
2 Department of Health (2000) *The NHS Plan: a plan for investment, a plan for reform.* Department of Health, London.
3 Jelley D and van Zwanenberg T (2000) Copying general practitioner referral letters to patients: a study of patients' views. *Br J Gen Pract.* **50**: 657–8.
4 Jelley D and van Zwanenberg T (2000) Peer appraisal in general practice: a descriptive study in the Northern Deanery. *Educ Gen Pract.* **11**: 281–7.
5 Whitford DL, Southern AJ, Braid E and Roberts SH (1995) Comprehensive diabetes care in North Tyneside. *Diabet Med.* **12**: 691–5.

PART 2

Clinical governance in practice

CHAPTER 5

What are patients looking for?

Marianne Rigge

This chapter describes how most patients are experts in their own right, and good judges of healthcare. PCTs need to develop skills to engage, understand and interpret the views of patients.

One of the most welcome statements in the present Government's original quality consultation paper, *A First-Class Service*, must surely have been 'We need to move away from merely counting numbers … clinical governance will help to ensure that quality resumes its rightful place at the heart of the NHS'.[1] Unfortunately the document failed to define quality. However, we *were* told, in the White Paper *The New NHS*, who the experts would be. 'Primary care professionals are identified as best placed to understand their patients' needs as a whole and to identify ways of making services more responsive'.[2] And the same document identified community health services as 'being able to take account of the special needs of black and ethnic minority patients and to draw attention to the wider health needs of the community'.

Five years on, we still remember, when putting together our response to the White Paper, being collectively dismayed by an editorial in the magazine *GP*, which clearly supported the idea that doctor knows best, while putting us silly patients firmly in our place. 'The public's grasp of complex health issues can be tenuous, and explaining the issues will absorb the time and resources of primary care groups. Those GPs involved in the process … are faced with the more pressing issues of commissioning care.'[3]

Other commentators went so far as to say that the patients' contribution in *The New NHS* had been relegated to a poor second or even third place, and that there was a real danger of signalling a return to the paternalistic attitudes that had been so heavily criticised in the past.[4]

The Government has now established the national Commission for Patient and Public Involvement in Health, with a raft of new local organisations – patient and public involvement forums and local authority Overview and Scrutiny Committees to replace the Community Health Councils as the local voice of the patient. It remains to be seen whether these new arrangements will perform better.

This chapter describes how most patients are experts in their own right – and good judges of the quality of healthcare. Primary care trusts need to develop skills to engage, understand and interpret the views of patients. It is clear that there is much to be done if patients' views and needs are to be genuinely taken on board, rather than being merely assumed by those who are deemed to know best.

The tokenistic appointment of sole lay representatives to primary care groups did not exactly suggest that we were going in the right direction. If we are to achieve a genuine engagement with users of health services as patients and carers, and as user representatives and advocates from the wealth of self-help and voluntary groups, we need first to acknowledge that many health professionals are unused to seeking out patients' views. Nor can we assume that even those who are willing to try will have the skills to engage, understand and correctly interpret those views.

How do you find out what makes a quality service from the patient's point of view? The answer is simple, although not simplistic. You ask the patient. Over the last decade or so, the College of Health has conducted well over 50 studies designed to find out about patients' views and experiences of virtually every aspect of the health service. We use a range of qualitative research techniques which we call 'consumer audit' – including, for example, focus groups. We have published a number of guides on how to go about this which have been commended by the NHS.[5-7] We offer training courses in qualitative research methods and in inclusive patient and public involvement as well as how to be effective in the role of lay non-executive member of a primary care trust (*see* section on sources of information and help).

What all of our studies have shown is that many patients are experts in their own right. They make good judges of the quality of every dimension of healthcare, including access and process, but most importantly outcome, as the following quotes from real patients demonstrate. They took part in a ground-breaking study conducted by the College of Health for the Royal College of Physicians to help to develop a methodology for producing patient-centred guidelines for rehabilitation after stroke.[8] We conducted a similar study with patients who had rheumatoid arthritis (RA).[9] The results of both studies suggest that GPs and the rest of the primary care team should be more alert to patients' needs for much better information, advice, support and guidance towards other sources of help to improve the quality of their lives. This could be a vastly important role for primary care trusts, but only if they find ways of tapping into the views and needs of their patients, as well as their unpaid carers – without whom the NHS would certainly collapse.

> The practice is very, very busy. Even with personal problems, you still feel you are being rushed in and rushed out as quickly as possible. It's very different from the practice I grew up with, where the family doctor knew the whole family and knew all of their problems. He was more of a friend.

Good communication, or the lack of it, are constantly recurring themes, as is the need for much more information.

> You'd phone the doctor any time you needed, and he came immediately. My husband was pretty ill. He still is. But if there's a problem, I know the doctor will come. He's very good. It's good to be able to talk to him

with all the problems ... he gives the time to listen ... he gives me good support.

(Stroke patient carer)

What's wrong is that doctors don't know enough about strokes or what it's like to be a stroke victim. You go to any surgery and they've got groups for diabetics, they've got groups for asthma, groups for arthritis. But there's no groups for stroke victims because the doctors don't know themselves. It took me years to find out about the Stroke Association, and when I think of all the help they could have given me when I really needed it, at my lowest ebb ...

(Stroke patient)

These attacks, they used to last for hours. They were very frightening and at the end I couldn't move. The doctor didn't seem to appreciate that I really was ill. All he could do was prescribe ever more steroids. ... But he retired and our new doctor referred me straight away and the rheumatologist was very stunned at the amount of steroids I'd had, and they'd done a lot of damage.

(RA patient)

One of the main lessons we have learned through such studies is that it is vital to let the patient or carer set the agenda, whether in a focus group or a one-to-one interview. This is especially the case with people from marginalised groups and those with special and complex needs, such as individuals with learning difficulties and mental health service users. They too are often faced with fragmented health and social services which do not necessarily talk to one another, despite all the rhetoric about seamless care.

Primary care trusts could really come into their own if they gave a proper place to meaningful involvement with their very different patient and client groups. Those best placed to orchestrate this may well not be GPs but, for instance, community psychiatric nurses and colleagues from other community and mental health services. Primary care trusts also need to think long and hard about the way some of their patients are typecast as 'heartsink' or as 'inappropriate attenders' at Accident and Emergency departments. The reality may be that it is their doctors who are heartsink – elderly, single-handed, working from substandard premises in dangerous parts of the inner city, where no one in their right mind would turn up hoping for a diagnosis of meningitis in their small child, or even the simplest treatment.

If there is a real window of opportunity to be grasped by the proposals set out in *The New NHS, A First-Class Service* and *The NHS Plan*, it must lie somewhere in the institution of primary care trusts, with strong primary care clinical governance committees.

The reason for this is that GPs and other members of the primary care team are not just the gatekeepers to the rest of the system – they also pick up the pieces. They hold the key to identifying the things that can go wrong when their patients fall between the different strands of the net of care. Despite improvements in waiting times, the College of Health still has a dossier of examples of the suffering that can be caused by the long periods that can elapse between referral to hospital and actually being treated by a consultant.[10]

During this time, they will be regarded as statistics to be counted, as trauma and orthopaedics or ophthalmology 'cases' – not as real people who may develop ulcers because they have to take so many painkillers for their arthritic hip or knee, or who fall and fracture their femur because they can no longer see properly.

It is the primary care team that will be the first port of call for patients in such need, and it is they who need to act as advocates on the patient's behalf. It is also the primary care team that is in a position to follow the patient pathway or journey through the health service, and then to link outcomes to the range of interventions and procedures they undergo, as well as the length of time they have to wait for them.

There is a challenge here for clinical governance committees – that they should start to pool resources and think big. If all primary care trusts were to agree to work with each other and genuinely share the information that they glean, including information about things that do not work as they should do, we could be well on the way to a revolution in the way in which the results of audit are put into practice. The National Patient Safety Agency could have an important role in helping with this.

However, one more step is needed. Primary care clinical governance committees need to work much more closely with patients, as well as with their colleagues in the acute sector, and to share the results of their work. This new partnership needs to be built into all of the systems set up for clinical governance. The unofficial jargon for this type of initiative is 'taking a whole systems approach'. In reality what it boils down to is intelligence and common sense, and patient groups are not lacking in either of these.

There still seems to be some kind of atavistic fear about sharing or publicising the results of audit. Of course, there are genuine and understandable reasons for clinicians to fear being identified when they are one among few (e.g. in a single primary healthcare team or acute service directorate), especially when litigation seems to be on the increase. And there is a corresponding and quite proper concern for patient confidentiality. However, that is the point. If clinical audit is shared and conducted on a much wider basis, there will be far less to fear in this respect. A more general point is that it is really not tenable to ask people to take part in research (and here I include audit) if you are not prepared to share with them even the generalisable results. This is particularly the case at a time of heightened public awareness following such tragic events as those that unfolded at the Bristol Royal Infirmary and Alder Hey Children's Hospital.

At the College of Health, we have a long-standing concern about the lack of information that is available to patients on consultants' qualifications, training and special interests. However, what is even more worrying is a growing trend for hospitals not to supply such information to GPs. In one of our surveys of every acute trust, we specifically asked for copies of information about consultants' special interests that they send to GPs. We were shocked to find that only 50% were supplying this information to GPs, never mind patients. The Freedom of Information Act 2000 places obligations on all NHS organisations, including general medical and dental practices. It has two main aspects:

- the right of any individual to make a request to a public authority for information and the duty of the public authority to reply to this request

- the placing of a duty on a public authority to publish information through a publication scheme.

Each NHS organisation was obliged to have a 'publication scheme' approved by the Information Commissioner by August 2003, and the individual's rights become effective in 2005. The challenge for primary care, from the patient's perspective, is to act in the spirit of the Act and not just to do the minimum necessary to get by.

If clinical governance is about anything, it must be about openness and accountability, and primary care trusts must insist on both if they are to play a major part in ironing out inefficiencies and inequalities in the system.

So what should primary care trusts be doing?

Take guidance from the National Institute for Clinical Excellence (NICE) and National Service Frameworks (NSFs) – but be proactive

- Put nationally agreed guidelines into practice by developing robust protocols for clinical audit at the local level, and involve patients and carers in the process.
- Make sure that patients and carers have access to patient versions of new guidelines as they are developed, and encourage them to be interactive about the ways in which these are put into practice and reported on.
- Enter into a continuing dialogue with trust clinical directorates to ensure that referral protocols are in place which conform with patient-centred guidelines.
- Agree with colleagues about what diagnostic and other tests should be ordered, by whom and at what stage, as well as how, when and by whom the results should be communicated to patients.
- Agree protocols for pain relief and other symptom management, especially for those patients who are unable to take analgesics for iatrogenic and other reasons.
- Be aware of the need to guide patients towards sources of information, help and advice for coping with their illness and its effects, especially if they have to wait for extended periods before treatment can be given. This might include physiotherapy and occupational therapy, aids and adaptations available through social services, welfare and other benefits, or self-help groups and voluntary organisations. You are not expected to know about all of these through some process of osmosis – there are others out there who do (*see* section on sources of information and help).
- Remember that many patients do not present with 'evidence-based illnesses'. You know better than most specialists that many illnesses are multifactorial in causation and presentation, and that some may never be satisfactorily diagnosed. This is not to say that patients do not need and deserve the best standard of treatment and management of the uncertainty to which this gives rise, which will probably be as distressing for you as it is for your patients. Certainly one of the downsides of the rapid rise in sub-specialisation is that there is now a dearth of the old-fashioned breed of physician whose wisdom and clinical judgement may not have been evidence based according to the new gold standards, but who remains much needed in 'difficult' cases.
- Insist on discharge protocols to ensure that patients receive the full range of information, advice and support that they need when they are sent home, and that you are fully informed about what has been done to them, by whom, and

what follow-up is planned. You also need to know what your patients have been told and what their expectations are.

• Follow through your patients and devise systems for reporting back on what happens to them after discharge. Otherwise your hospital colleagues will not know what the final outcomes really were. Seeing a junior doctor in outpatients six weeks after discharge will not suffice. They are likely to be ticked off as a 'successful outcome' because they have been discharged alive and have managed to get to their postoperative appointment in one piece! In some general practices the reception staff routinely phone patients immediately after they have been discharged from hospital to check that they are all right (*see* Chapter 4).

• Bear in mind that a rigid insistence that guidelines must be based only on the evidence of scientific trials is unhelpful to patients. Medicine is an art as well as a science, and sometimes results will depend as much on patient compliance as on the treatment administered. This in turn may depend on the quality of communication with patients and the information that they are given. Your hospital colleagues may fall short on this. It is not necessarily their fault, as they will probably not have been taught much about this in medical school, and almost certainly not thereafter.

• Do not believe everything they say about randomised controlled trials being the gold standard. Vast numbers of procedures and treatments that are being carried out on your patients have never been subjected to these trials – and for some it would not be possible. In any case, there is a recognised bias towards reporting only the results of those trials that have been successful, and most of these will have ruled out individuals who might 'spoil' the science because they are children, women of childbearing age, elderly, come from ethnic minorities or have other things the matter with them.

• Remember that an over-reliance on evidence-based guidelines may mean that patients who are suffering from conditions or undergoing treatments for which there is a lack of scientifically robust data are denied information about what is current good or acceptable practice in the 'light' of known uncertainty.

Where do we go from here?

NICE may be part of the answer, but it will not be a panacea. At the present rate of guideline development, we are many years away from being able to tell patients who are suffering from even some of the most common conditions what sort of standard of treatment they should be able to expect. Where there is confusion and uncertainty, they deserve to be told that. What is needed is a more pragmatic and patient-centred approach. The people who are best placed to take that approach are those whom patients approach in the first place – the ones in whom they put their trust in what remains an intrinsically personal and most favoured relationship. They do not deserve to be let down by squabbles about who should have most power in the new systems that are being imposed on this 'new' NHS of ours; because it is all of ours, and the ethos of compassion and care needs to prevail if we are to make the best of it. That is what patients are looking for from clinical governance in primary healthcare.

Sources of information and help

College of Health training, research and consultancy for effective patient and public involvement

The College of Health offers a range of training workshops promoting effective patient and public involvement. They include training in a range of research and consultation methods, as well as guidance on patient and public involvement policy and practice. We also offer training to support lay representatives in health and social care.

Training can also be run at your site, as well as in London and other major cities, and can be tailored to your specific needs.

The College's research team conducts a range of research and consultation projects with both users and professionals to enable health and social care organisations to be more responsive to the needs and views of users.

For further information about our training and research services, please contact:

The College of Health
St Margaret's House
21 Old Ford Road
London E2 9PL
Tel: 020 8983 1225/1553
Email: info@collegeofhealth.org.uk

Self-help group database

Health Data 2000
This database, programmed in Microsoft Access, contains details of over 2000 national health-related self-help groups.

Local health and self-help groups shell
The Health Data 2000 Self-Help Groups database can be provided with a shell to populate with your own local health information, including local groups, health authority details, primary care details, NHS trusts, opticians, dentists, community pharmacies, clinics, etc.

Health information

Healthline tapes
The College of Health has produced over 500 audio tapes on health-related topics. Professionally recorded, they are designed to be listened to over the phone and are thus available 24 hours a day. The information is regularly updated and validated by medical experts.

Healthline factsheets

Factsheets on over 500 health-related topics can be printed out from your computer to provide another valuable information resource for your patients. Using a question-and-answer format, the factsheets provide important basic information, often including further sources of health advice and support.

Practical points

- Patients and carers are good judges of the quality of healthcare.
- There are well-described techniques for ascertaining the views of patients.
- Primary care trusts should pool resources and share information so that the results of audit are put into practice.
- Involve patients and carers in the process of implementing national guidelines, and make sure that they have patient versions of the guidelines.
- Work with secondary care clinicians and patients to sort out referral and discharge protocols.
- Guide patients towards sources of information, help and advice. These sources do exist. Primary care practitioners do not have to know it all.
- Many patients do not have 'evidence-based illnesses', but they still deserve the best standard of treatment, care and compassion.

References

1 Department of Health (1998) *A First-Class Service: quality in the new NHS*. Department of Health, London.

2 Department of Health (1997) *The New NHS: modern, dependable*. The Stationery Office, London.

3 Editorial (1998) Care needed with patient input. *Gen Practitioner*. **16 January**.

4 Rhodes P and Nocon A (1998) *User Involvement and the NHS Reforms: health expectations*. Blackwell Science, Oxford.

5 College of Health (1994) *Consumer Audit Guidelines*. College of Health, London.

6 Kelson M (1995) *Consumer Involvement Initiatives in Clinical Audit and Outcomes: a review of developments and issues in the identification of good practice*. College of Health, London.

7 Kelson M (1999) *Patient-Defined Outcomes*. Paper prepared on behalf of the Clinical Outcomes Group Patient Group. College of Health, London.

8 Kelson M, Rigge M and Ford C (1998) *Report on a College of Health and Royal College of Physicians Project: stroke rehabilitation patient and carer views*. Royal College of Physicians, London.

9 Rigge M (1998) Developing patient-centred guidelines for rheumatoid arthritis. *Guidelines Pract.* **1**: 25–8.

10 Rigge M (1998) *College of Health Response to the NHS Consultative Paper: The New NHS: guidance on out-of-area treatment*. College of Health, London.

CHAPTER 6

Evidence-based practice

Ian Watt

This chapter describes a structured approach to evidence-based practice. This approach includes five steps – asking questions, tracking down the evidence, appraising the evidence, applying evidence-based practice and evaluating performance.

What is evidence-based practice?

Evidence-based healthcare is one of the key components of clinical governance. Unfortunately, the term has slipped into everyday usage with little common understanding of what it involves. Many misconceptions and prejudices have arisen around evidence-based practice, and those involved in clinical governance will need to overcome them.

Although the philosophical origins of evidence-based practice have been said to date back to mid-nineteenth century Paris and earlier, it is only since the early 1990s that its importance has been emphasised in the NHS. In 1991, the NHS Research and Development Strategy was launched to 'secure a knowledge-based health service in which clinical, managerial and policy decisions are based on sound and pertinent information'. Since then, a number of different initiatives have been used to promote what has essentially been the same concept – evidence-based practice. Given the plethora of terms in use, it is worth clarifying definitions here.

Sackett and colleagues have defined evidence-based medicine as 'the conscientious, explicit and judicious use of current best evidence in making decisions about the care of individual patients'[1]. They go on to state that this means 'integrating individual clinical expertise with the best available external clinical evidence from systematic research. This should be done in consultation with the patient in order to decide upon the option which suits that patient best'.

One of the criticisms that has been levelled at evidence-based medicine is that it leads to so-called 'cookbook medicine'. As defined above, however, there is a clear recognition of the importance of clinical expertise and individual patient factors in deciding whether and how external evidence should be applied to an individual. Slavish 'cookbook' approaches to individual patient care should be discouraged. Following on from the definition given by Sackett and colleagues, the term 'evidence-based' has been applied to a number of areas in health and healthcare (e.g. nursing, health promotion and policy making). For simplicity, the generic term 'evidence-based practice' is used here.

Another term that is sometimes used interchangeably with evidence-based practice is clinical effectiveness. Formal definitions are given in Box 6.1, but more simply, an effective healthcare intervention can be defined as one that does more good than harm, and a cost-effective intervention can be defined as one that does more good than harm at least cost.

Box 6.1 Some definitions

Evidence-based practice
The conscientious, explicit and judicious use of current best evidence in making decisions about the care of individual patients.

Effectiveness
The extent to which a specific intervention, procedure, regimen or service, when deployed in the field, does what it is intended to do for a defined population.

Efficacy
The extent to which a specific intervention, procedure, regimen or service produces a beneficial result under ideal conditions. Ideally, the determination of efficacy is based on the results of a randomised controlled trial.

An approach to evidence-based practice

As evidence-based practice has developed, a more formal approach to its application has gained acceptance. This proposes five steps whereby answers to clinical questions are sought, appraised and applied in clinical practice (*see* Box 6.2).[2]

For the individual practitioner, evidence-based practice provides one approach to self-directed learning, where answers can be found for the diagnostic, prognostic and therapeutic problems presented by patients. Evidence-based practice also offers a framework for those practitioners with a responsibility for the quality of healthcare at a population level. For example, those involved in developing a clinical protocol, or guideline, for a primary care trust should seek to ensure that it is based on good evidence.

Box 6.2 Steps in evidence-based practice[2]

What does evidence-based practice involve?
1 Converting information needs into answerable questions
2 Tracking down the best evidence with which to answer them
3 Critically appraising that evidence for its validity (closeness to the truth) and usefulness (clinical applicability)
4 Applying the results of this appraisal to clinical practice
5 Evaluating performance

Although the steps outlined in Box 6.2 may appear overly rigid and time-consuming, they do provide a structured framework for the application of evidence in clinical practice. Not all of them have to be undertaken by the same person. Each of the stages will now be considered in more detail.

Stage 1: asking questions

Clinical questions arise from individual clinical encounters and from the process of developing clinical policies and guidance. Practitioners may overestimate the extent and accuracy of their clinical knowledge, and are not always aware of the latest research findings. Inevitably, knowledge and probably clinical performance deteriorate with time. To prevent this, practitioners need to be prepared to reflect on their practice and question its appropriateness. Without this reflection, practice fails to benefit from research and risks becoming out of date, leading to suboptimal care for patients.

The process of clinical governance will need to ensure that practitioners can question their practice, and that effective lifelong learning is encouraged and supported. Evidence-based practice starts by identifying information needs and converting these into answerable questions. Often this is not as easy as it sounds. If questions are poorly constructed and/or too vague, it may not be possible to find the best evidence with which to answer them. To help focus such questions, they should be based on the following four components:

1 the patient or problem
2 the intervention
3 the comparison intervention (if relevant)
4 the outcomes of interest.

For example:

1 in obese patients with type 2 diabetes…
2 does metformin…
3 compared with sulphonylureas…
4 lead to improved diabetic control, lower all-cause mortality and improve quality of life?

Stage 2: tracking down the evidence

Evidence, in a legal sense, may come from a number of sources. However, in the context of evidence-based practice it should ideally come from high-quality scientific research. The most appropriate type of research study from which to glean the evidence will vary according to the nature of the question that is posed. For example, a question concerning the effectiveness of an intervention is normally best answered by a randomised controlled trial. This is because randomised controlled trials, if performed well, are the research design that is least susceptible to bias.

Even when undertaken correctly, some study designs are more susceptible to bias than others. For this reason, hierarchies of evidence have been developed to help make judgements about the strength of the evidence available. One such hierarchy is shown in Box 6.3, with the most reliable designs (with respect to answering questions of effectiveness) at the top. The least reliable evidence on clinical effectiveness comes from expert opinion.

Box 6.3   Hierarchy of evidence

1 Evidence from systematic reviews of multiple, well-designed, randomised controlled trials
2 Evidence from at least one properly designed, randomised controlled trial of appropriate size
3 Evidence from well-designed, non-randomised trials, non-controlled intervention studies, cohort studies, time series or case–control studies
4 Evidence from well-designed, non-experimental studies from more than one centre or research group
5 Opinions of respected authorities based on clinical experience, descriptive studies and reports of expert committees

---

This is not to imply that randomised controlled trials can be used to answer all healthcare questions. For example, they may not always be feasible because of cost or ethical considerations.

Another research design which is useful in evidence-based practice is the systematic review (*see* Box 6.4).[3] Systematic reviews differ from ordinary reviews in following an explicit method and seeking to be as objective as possible. Given the increasing amount of new research evidence (over 2 000 000 articles published annually in over 20 000 biomedical journals), systematic reviews can provide reliable summaries of research evidence, and are particularly useful for busy practitioners in primary care.

Box 6.4   Systematic reviews[3]

Review
The general term for all attempts to synthesise the results and conclusions of two or more publications on a given topic.

Systematic review
A comprehensive review which strives to identify and track down all of the literature on a topic (also called a systematic literature review).

Meta-analysis
A technique which incorporates a specific statistical strategy for assembling the results of several studies into a single estimated overall result.

Sources of evidence

It is a salutary fact that only a small proportion of the vast quantity of research which is published each year is of high quality. In addition, the reliable evidence may be scattered across many different journals. Electronic databases such as Medline and Embase can help to identify relevant studies, but searching these databases is not always easy. Because of inadequacies in the indexing of research papers, even the best searchers may fail to find relevant studies. In general, only about half of the randomised controlled trials in Medline can be found by even the best electronic searcher.[4] In addition, electronic databases are not exhaustive in their coverage. For example, Medline covers only about 6000 of the 20 000 journals that are published worldwide.

Potential solutions to these problems include the following:

- using good search strategies
- seeking systematic reviews to answer questions
- using specialised databases.

The help of an experienced librarian is often invaluable.

Search strategies

The identification of relevant research to meet a specific information need can be optimised by using a tailored set of instructions for a particular database, in order to give the richest yield of relevant studies. Information on designing effective search strategies is given in Box 6.5.

Box 6.5   Helpful information on search strategies

Electronic sources of advice
Predefined search strategies to locate systematic reviews on Medline and CINAHL are available at the website of the NHS Centre for Reviews and Dissemination: www.york.ac.uk/inst/crd/search.htm

A range of strategies, including search strategies to locate randomised controlled trials, can be found at http://www.minervation.com/cebm

Search strategies are available via the PubMED free Medline site: www.ncbi. nlm.nih.gov/PubMed/clinical.html

Further reading
- Muir Gray JA (2001) *Evidence-Based Healthcare*. Churchill Livingstone, Edinburgh.
- Glanville J (1999) Carrying out the literature search. In: S Curran and CJ Williams (eds) *Clinical Research in Psychiatry*. Butterworth-Heinemann, Oxford.

Systematic reviews

Because good systematic reviews will have tracked down and appraised most of the relevant high-quality research on a specific area of concern, they undoubtedly represent the best starting point for answering clinical questions. In the past, good systematic reviews were few and far between. However, they are now becoming an increasingly popular research tool applied to a wide range of clinical areas, and their quality is also improving.

Perhaps the most influential group in this respect is the Cochrane Collaboration – an international research initiative that was set up to produce, maintain and disseminate systematic reviews of the research evidence relevant to health and healthcare. Cochrane Reviews can be found in the Cochrane Library (*see* Box 6.6) – a regularly updated electronic library of related databases.

Box 6.6   Helpful sources of systematic reviews

The Cochrane Library
This is a regularly updated electronic library containing the following:

- the Cochrane Database of Systematic Reviews – full text of reviews produced and updated by the Cochrane Collaboration
- the Database of Abstracts of Reviews of Effectiveness (DARE) produced by the NHS Centre for Reviews and Dissemination, University of York – contains structured summaries of quality-assessed reviews produced by non-Cochrane researchers
- the Cochrane Controlled Trials Register – a bibliography of over 100 000 controlled trials
- the Cochrane Review Methodology Database – a bibliography of articles on undertaking systematic reviews
- the NHS Economic Evaluation Database – structured summaries of economic evaluations; available free online, and also on the Cochrane Library.

The Cochrane Library is available via the National electronic Library for Health (access is free to UK users at www.nelh.nhs.uk), as a CD-ROM, or via Internet subscription (details are available at www.cochrane.org).

The NHS Centre for Reviews and Dissemination (NHS CRD), University of York
This is a facility commissioned by the NHS Research and Development Programme to undertake, commission and identify reviews on the effectiveness and cost-effectiveness of health interventions, and disseminate them to the NHS. It produces the following:

- DARE – *see* above (also free online)
- *Effective Health Care Bulletin* – a bimonthly bulletin in which the effectiveness of a variety of healthcare interventions is examined, based on a systematic review and synthesis of research on clinical effectiveness, cost-effectiveness and acceptability. It is widely distributed free of charge throughout the NHS, including all general practices and postgraduate libraries.

- *Effectiveness Matters* – bulletins containing short summaries of systematic reviews with important messages for the NHS. They have a similar distribution to the *Effective Health Care Bulletin*.

Information on CRD or its products can be obtained from the University of York, York YO1 5DD. Email: revdis@york.ac.uk.
CRD databases can be searched via their web pages at:
http://nhscrd.york.ac.uk/welcome.html

Also in the Cochrane Library (and available online in its own right) is another source of high-quality systematic reviews, namely the Database of Abstracts of Reviews of Effectiveness (DARE). This is produced by the NHS Centre for Reviews and Dissemination (NHS CRD) at the University of York, and consists of abstracts of quality-assessed systematic reviews, together with critical commentaries written by York researchers. CRD also produced a similar database of economic evaluations – the NHS Economic Evaluation Database (NHS EED) – which can be used to help answer questions related to cost-effectiveness.

Specialist databases

Medline is probably the electronic database that is most familiar to health professionals, and it is a useful resource. However, because of the problems of limited coverage of published journals and inadequate indexing of research papers, it may not be the most effective way of meeting specialised information needs or finding specific types of research, such as systematic reviews. Therefore it is always worth asking a librarian about the existence of databases specialising in research in the specified area of interest. With regard to specific types of research study (e.g. randomised controlled trials and systematic reviews), the Cochrane Library should normally be the first database to be consulted.

Stage 3: appraising the evidence

Having tracked down the research information, the next step is to assess its validity (i.e. to make an assessment of how 'true' the study conclusions are). Two aspects of validity are normally assessed, namely *internal validity* (how likely it is that the study conclusions are biased due to inadequacies in study design or analysis), and *external validity* (reliability; how far the study conclusions can be generalised to circumstances other than those found in the original research).

It is beyond the scope of this chapter to provide detailed advice on the assessment of the validity of research studies. However, it is important to stress that research conclusions should not be adopted without some appraisal of the studies from which they have been drawn. Such appraisal is often helped by following a checklist of questions so that all of the important issues of design, analysis and interpretation can be assessed. Sources of advice on critical appraisal, including useful checklists, are listed in Box 6.7.

Box 6.7 Some examples of helpful information on critical appraisal

- Crombie IK (1996) *The Pocket Guide to Critical Appraisal*. BMJ Publishing, London.
- Sackett DL, Haynes RB, Guyatt GTT *et al.* (1991) *Clinical Epidemiology*. Little Brown, Boston, MA.
- Users' Guides to the Medical Literature prepared by the Evidence-Based Medicine Working Group are available on the Internet at: www.cche.net/usersguides/main.asp
- *How to Read a Paper* – a series of articles written by T Greenhalgh that provide a good overview of basic critical appraisal. Published in the *British Medical Journal* in eight weekly articles (starting *BMJ*. (1997) **315**: 180–3) and also now available in a book: Greenhalgh T (2000) *How to Read a Paper*. BMJ Publishing, London.
- Chambers R (1998) *Clinical Effectiveness Made Easy: first thoughts on clinical governance*. Radcliffe Medical Press, Oxford.
- Sackett DL, Straus SE, Scott Richardson W *et al.* (2000) *Evidence-Based Medicine: how to practise and teach EBM*. Churchill Livingstone, Edinburgh.

Increasingly there are now sources of research-based information becoming available where someone else has appraised the validity of the studies. These assessments, undertaken by individuals with expertise in critical appraisal, are useful for busy practitioners who may have neither the time nor the skills to undertake detailed appraisals themselves.

Some examples of sources of appraised research information are listed in Box 6.8. As already indicated, systematic reviews are useful in this respect, as the reviewer will have had to appraise all of the relevant primary research. Unfortunately, systematic reviews can also be prone to bias, like any other research method, and should not be interpreted uncritically.

Box 6.8 Some examples of sources of appraised research evidence

- *Evidence-Based Medicine* – a bimonthly journal which identifies and appraises high-quality, clinically relevant research. The articles are summarised in informative abstracts and commented on by clinical experts. For further information, *see* http://ebm.bmjjournals.com/
- *ACP Journal Club* – related to *Evidence-Based Medicine* and published by the American College of Physicians. Abstracts are restricted to internal medicine: www.acpjc.org/
- *Evidence-Based Nursing*: http://ebn.bmjjournals.com/
- *Evidence-Based Mental Health*: http://ebmh.bmjjournals.com/
- *Evidence-Based Health Care*: www.harcourt-international.com/journals/ebhc/
- *Bandolier* – a monthly newsletter published by the NHS. It aims to produce up-to-date information on the effectiveness of healthcare interventions: www.jr2.ox.ac.uk/Bandolier

- *Drug and Therapeutics Bulletin* – an independent review of the effectiveness of mainly pharmacological interventions, produced by the Consumers' Association: www.which.net/health/dtb/main.html
- *Clinical Evidence* – a twice-yearly compendium of evidence on the benefits and adverse effects of common clinical interventions: www.clinicalevidence.com

These and other information sources are also available via the National electronic Library for Health (www.nelh.nhs.uk) – an electronic library for NHS staff, patients and the public.

Stage 4: applying evidence-based practice

For clinical governance to succeed, the principles at least behind the steps outlined above will need to be understood by all primary care staff. Given that this will not be achieved easily, it is reasonable to ask 'why bother?'. Three main reasons can be given.

1 Medical knowledge is changing at a rapid rate. The notion that the body of knowledge acquired by completion of professional training remains unchanged throughout a clinical career is simply untenable.
2 The sheer volume of health-related research and the wide variation in its quality makes it increasingly easy to miss valid research that could benefit patient care.
3 Patients are becoming much better informed about all aspects of their healthcare through sources such as magazines, television and, more recently, the Internet.

Although the information that patients gather may not always be valid, they do want to discuss the options for their healthcare, and they expect their practitioners to be well informed. The rationale for evidence-based practice is thus well founded, but its widespread application in primary care raises a number of issues.

Finding the time and other resources

Almost every clinical encounter generates the need for further information for the practitioner. In addition, clinical guidelines are becoming increasingly popular in the drive to improve the quality of healthcare. There is a danger that practitioners could become swamped by the process of tracking down, appraising and applying the answers to all of their clinical questions. For most clinicians, time is the major barrier and they will need to prioritise their information needs. Busy clinicians may find the following criteria helpful:

- the importance of the question to the patient's care
- the feasibility of answering the question in the time available
- the interest of the clinician in the problem
- the questions that are most likely to provide answers which help other patients.

Those charged with the development of evidence-based guidelines will also need to prioritise the topics addressed. If primary care is overloaded with guidelines, they will not be implemented effectively, but will be left to gather dust on some forgotten shelf.

In addition to time, evidence-based practice also requires access to relevant sources of research information. A good postgraduate library service is important, but it is no substitute for decent resources at practice level. Practices need to have good information facilities of their own. In particular, they should have access to electronic media, such as the Internet, and to databases, such as the Cochrane Library. The Cochrane Library is available via the National electronic Library for Health (www.nelh.nhs.uk) – an electronic library for NHS staff, patients and the public.

A lack of evidence

Primary care practitioners see an extremely wide range of clinical problems and presentations. One consequence of this is that the research which is needed to answer a particular clinical question may not have been undertaken. Even where the research exists, it may have been undertaken in circumstances that caution against its application in primary care. To safeguard internal validity, researchers often control the types of patients who are recruited to studies.

For example, a study of the efficacy of a new antihypertensive drug might include only men aged under 65 years with no comorbidities. This makes it difficult to generalise the study conclusions to the wide variety of patients who are seen in primary care. There are further problems of generalisability. Much of the research is undertaken in secondary care, where the patients do not necessarily have the same characteristics as those with the same condition in the wider community.

However, these issues should not prevent evidence-based practice from being carried out in primary care. They highlight the need for a critical approach, and for more research to be undertaken in primary care. And there still remains a large volume of evidence that can be usefully applied in the primary care setting.[5]

The public

The public is becoming better informed about many aspects of healthcare. This can act as a spur to evidence-based practice, particularly when patients want an informed discussion about their care. The discussion of research evidence with lay people inevitably requires a certain skill to explain and interpret the findings. Practitioners need to gauge patients' level of understanding, the amount of information they require and their desired level of involvement in decision making. Much of the publicly accessible health information is of good quality, but some of it is not. Practitioners may need to appraise information jointly with the patient. An informed public should not be viewed as a threat, although it does make it harder for practitioners to avoid taking an evidence-based approach.

Stage 5: evaluating performance

The final part of the evidence-based practice pathway involves assessing whether research recommendations have been implemented, and what impact they have had on patients' outcomes. For the individual practitioner, a formal evaluation of whether the answers to all clinical questions assessed by this approach are implemented would be a daunting task. Nevertheless, this step emphasises that practical recommendations are rarely implemented without a conscious strategy.

In addition, once implemented, the improved patient outcomes predicted by the original research may not be realised if there are differences between the study conditions and practice. Practitioners should at least undertake regular informal evaluations of their implementation of evidence-based practice.

A number of more formal methods of monitoring performance are discussed elsewhere in this book (*see* Chapters 8 and 9). Clinical audit is probably the best known of these methods, and audit criteria and standards should be based on best evidence. Formal mechanisms to evaluate performance need to be restricted to priority topics, particularly those where large groups of patients might benefit.

Conclusion

This chapter has provided a brief overview of the rationale, methods and issues surrounding evidence-based practice. For many in primary care, the message of evidence-based practice is neither new nor surprising. Good practitioners have always sought to keep their practice up to date. The processes of clinical governance should help all in primary care in their application of evidence-based practice.

Practical points

- Evidence-based practice is not new.
- It concerns the use of current best evidence in the care of individual patients.
- There are vast amounts of published research, not all of which is of good quality.
- Evidence-based practice provides a structured approach to finding, appraising and applying best evidence.
- There are useful sources of summarised research evidence for busy practitioners.
- The help of a good librarian can be invaluable.
- Primary care teams should have access to the Internet and the Cochrane Library.
- Patients are becoming increasingly better informed, and practitioners need to be able to discuss the evidence with them.

References

1 Sackett DL, Rosenberg WMC, Gray JAM *et al*. (1996) Evidence-based medicine: what it is and what it isn't. *BMJ*. **312**: 71–2.
2 Sackett DL, Richardson WS, Rosenberg W *et al*. (1997) *Evidence-Based Medicine*. Churchill Livingstone, Edinburgh.

3 Chalmers I and Altman DG (eds) (1995) *Systematic Reviews*. BMJ Publishing, London.
4 Muir Gray JA (1997) *Evidence-Based Healthcare: how to make health policy and management decisions*. Churchill Livingstone, Edinburgh.
5 Gill P, Dowell AC, Neal RP *et al*. (1996) Evidence-based general practice: a retrospective study of interventions in our training practice. *BMJ*. **312**: 819–21.

CHAPTER 7

Disseminating and implementing evidence-based practice

Martin Eccles, Jeremy Grimshaw and Robbie Foy

This chapter analyses the effectiveness of a range of interventions which are used to bring about changes in clinical behaviour. No single intervention is effective under all circumstances. Multifaceted approaches targeted at one behaviour may be more likely to succeed, but are also more costly.

Introduction

In all healthcare systems there is an increasing awareness of the need for quality assurance for the following reasons.

- The resources available for healthcare are limited.
- The variations in clinical practice are unexplained by characteristics of patients, their illnesses or the setting of care.
- There is evidence of unacceptable standards of practice.
- There is a lag between the emergence of research evidence and its incorporation into routine practice.

All of this is set against a background of demand for increasing professional and managerial accountability.

In response to such issues, professional bodies emphasised professionals' responsibilities to ensure quality of care (e.g. Royal College of General Practitioners[1]) and issued guidelines (e.g. Royal College of Radiologists[2]). In addition, a range of policy initiatives encouraged and supported quality assurance activities, such as the introduction of clinical audit,[3] the clinical effectiveness initiative[4] and the NHS Research and Development (R&D) Programme.[5] Yet the impact of these earlier initiatives was undermined by significant organisational shortcomings. For example, clinical audit often appeared to be an *ad hoc* activity led by clinicians in isolation from the rest of the organisation (and sometimes even from their peers).[6] There was a lack of a broader framework to ensure that the emphasis of clinical audit shifted from measuring performance and providing small amounts of feedback towards changing practice. Secondly, the dissemination of clinical guidelines and rapid expansion in the availability of other paper and electronic sources of information were seldom accompanied by active local implementation. Clinical governance united these and other policy initiatives.[7]

Clinical governance is described as an initiative which includes action to ensure that 'good practice is rapidly disseminated and systems are in place to ensure continuous improvements in clinical care'.[7] If the clinical effectiveness element of clinical governance is to achieve its potential, and quality assurance and implementation activities are to be effective in improving the care that patients receive, there are two key steps. The first of these is the rapid identification of effective treatments and healthcare interventions, and the second step is the use of effective dissemination and implementation strategies to encourage the adoption of these effective interventions in routine practice.[8]

Identifying effective treatments and healthcare interventions

Over 20 000 medical journals are published each year, containing research papers of variable quality and relevance. However, the average time that an NHS consultant has available to read is about one hour a week. It is clearly impossible for healthcare professionals to keep up to date with primary research. To overcome this problem, Guyatt and Rennie suggest 'that resolving a clinical problem begins with a search for a valid overview or practice guideline as the most efficient method of deciding on the best patient care'.[9] The issues of locating evidence are covered in Chapter 6. However, a number of points are worth emphasising here.

First, the best starting place when looking for systematic reviews is the Cochrane Library (www.cochrane.de). Box 7.1 summarises the Library contents. Together these represent the most comprehensive starting place for searching for clinical trials and high-quality systematic reviews.[10]

Box 7.1 The Cochrane Library: contents of Issue 4 in 2002

- Cochrane Database of Systematic Reviews, including 1519 complete reviews and 1136 protocols for reviews undertaken by members of the collaboration
- Cochrane Controlled Trials Register of almost 350 000 trials
- Database of Abstracts of Reviews of Effectiveness, including 2940 abstracts
- NHS Economic Evaluation Database, containing 3842 critically appraised economic evaluations
- Cochrane Review Methodology Database

Secondly, finding high-quality clinical guidelines can be problematic. Guidelines are often published in the 'grey' literature and are not indexed in the commonly available bibliographic databases (although a number of bibliographic databases are available that specialise in 'grey' literature). For example, none of the guidelines published by the Agency for Healthcare Research and Quality (AHRQ) can be found on Medline. Even when guidelines are published in indexed journals, the best search strategies have yet to be developed. In the Ovid version of Medline, practice guidelines can be identified under a variety of headings, including *guideline* (publication type), *practice guideline* (publication type), *practice guidelines* (MeSH heading), *Consensus Development Conference* (publication type) and *Consensus Development Conference, NIH* (publication type). A preliminary examination across several clinical areas suggests that *guideline* (publication type) is probably the most sensitive and specific single search term.

Fortunately, there are other resources available to help practitioners. In particular, there are a number of sites on the Internet which catalogue clinical guidelines. For example, the AHRQ-funded Guideline Clearing House has details of 974 guideline summaries produced by a diverse range of organisations. Such sites are becoming the best source for identifying full text versions or abstracts of guidelines (*see* Box 7.2).

Box 7.2   Electronic guideline resources

National Guidelines Clearing House – US Agency for Healthcare Research and Quality funded site which includes index of clinical practice guidelines, structured abstracts of guidelines and comparisons of guidelines for the same clinical topic (www.guidelines.gov)
National Institute for Clinical Excellence – website of UK organisation with responsibility for commissioning guidelines (www.nice.org.uk)
Scottish Intercollegiate Guidelines Network (SIGN) – full text copies of SIGN guidelines (www.show.scot.nhs.uk/sign/index.html)
Canadian Medical Association Clinical Practice Guidelines Infobase – index of clinical practice guidelines, includes downloadable full text versions or abstracts for most guidelines (www.cma.ca/cpgs/index.html)
New Zealand Guidelines Group – full text versions of some guidelines, as well as other useful guideline-related resources (www.nzgg.org.nz/library.cfm)

Note: at the time of writing the electronic addresses given are correct. However, they are liable to change over time.

Another strategy that primary care staff could consider is to develop a practice library of valid clinical guidelines by appraising any guidelines they are sent. In recent years, clinicians have been overwhelmed by a proliferation of guidelines,[11] frequently of unreliable quality. Checklists have been designed to help practitioners to appraise guidelines (e.g. by Cluzeau and colleagues[12]).

Evidence-based implementation

There is an increasing awareness that active implementation strategies are required if new evidence is to be routinely incorporated into practice. However, most of the approaches to changing clinical practice are more often based on beliefs than on scientific evidence. This leads to the proposition that 'evidence-based medicine should be complemented by evidence-based implementation'.[13]

As with clinical care, systematic reviews of rigorous studies can contribute greatly to our knowledge about what works in changing professional and organisational behaviour. The Cochrane Effective Practice and Organisation of Care (EPOC) Group undertakes systematic reviews of behavioural/professional educational, organisational, financial and regulatory interventions to improve professional practice and the delivery of effective health services.[14] Members of this group undertook an overview of systematic reviews of professional behaviour change strategies,[15] a summary of which is provided below. In total, 44 systematic reviews fulfilled the inclusion criteria, of which 34 reviews had been published since 1994. This overview suggested that it was possible to identify strategies that were either more or less effective. Notably, the included reviews were generally of poor quality and frequently ignored common methodological weaknesses in primary studies.

As with clinical research, new knowledge is continually emerging about what works in changing professional behaviour. More recently, we undertook a systematic review of rigorous evaluations of guideline dissemination and implementation strategies, funded by the NHS Health Technology Assessment (HTA) Programme.[16] This review covered studies published up to 1998, and represents the most comprehensive systematic review to date, including 235 studies reporting 309 different comparisons. Interestingly, it challenges some of the conclusions of previous reviews. A summary of the overview of systematic reviews is presented here, complemented by relevant findings of the HTA review.

Broad strategies

The overview identified 15 reviews focusing on broad strategies (involving a variety of strategies targeting a variety of behaviours), including continuing medical education (CME), dissemination and implementation of guidelines, and programmes to enhance the quality and economy of primary care.

Continuing medical education

Davis and colleagues identified 99 studies involving 160 comparisons of CME interventions.[17] Improvements in at least one major end point were identified in 68% of studies. Single interventions that were likely to be effective included educational outreach, opinion leaders, patient-mediated interventions and reminders. These are described later in this chapter. Multifaceted interventions and those interventions where the potential barriers were assessed in advance were more likely to be successful.

The introduction of clinical guidelines

A review of passive dissemination of consensus recommendations concluded that there was little evidence that it alone resulted in behaviour change.[18] A later review of factors which influenced compliance with guideline recommendations found that compliance was lower for recommendations that were more complex.[19] In 1994, the *Effective Health Care Bulletin* reviewed studies that evaluated the introduction of guidelines.[20] In 81 of 89 studies, improved compliance with guideline recommendations was reported, and improvements in patient outcome were seen in 12 of 17 studies that measured outcome. The *Bulletin* authors concluded that guidelines can change clinical practice. Guidelines were more likely to be effective if they took account of local circumstances, were disseminated by active educational interventions and were implemented by patient-specific reminders. There was inconclusive evidence as to whether guidelines developed by the 'end users' (local guidelines) were more likely to be effective than guidelines developed without their involvement (national guidelines). In another review of 102 studies of interventions to improve the delivery of healthcare services, it was observed that dissemination on its own resulted in little or no change in behaviour.[21] Furthermore, more complex interventions, although frequently effective, usually produced only moderate effects. The authors concluded that there are 'no magic bullets' for clinical behaviour change. There is a range of interventions that can lead to change, but no single intervention is always effective.

Similarly, a review of the effectiveness of introducing guidelines in primary care settings identified 61 studies, which showed considerable variation in the effectiveness of a range of interventions.[22] Multifaceted interventions combining more than one intervention are more likely to be effective, but may be more expensive. One review of studies evaluating the introduction of guidelines for professions allied to medicine (PAMS) found only 18 studies, of generally poor quality.[23] There was insufficient evidence to determine the effectiveness of different strategies, although a number of studies suggested that guidelines could be used to support the extension of nursing roles.

In summary, there are examples of programmes that have been successful in improving aspects of primary care, but there remain significant gaps in our knowledge about what works best.[24]

Interventions to improve specific behaviours

Other reviews have focused on interventions that target specific behaviours – for example, preventive care, prescribing, referrals and test ordering.

Preventive care

A number of reviews have examined a range of interventions that are used to influence all aspects of prevention. One study found improvements in the process of care in 28 of 32 studies.[25] However, significant improvements in the outcome of care were present in only four of the 13 studies that measured outcome. In primary care a range of effective interventions has been identified, with multifaceted interventions including reminders emerging as the most effective.[26] However, such interventions may incur greater cost, and they need to be focused rather than employed with a shotgun approach.[27]

Prescribing

To improve prescribing, mailed educational materials alone are generally ineffective.[28] Educational outreach approaches and ongoing feedback are usually effective, but there is insufficient evidence to determine the effectiveness of reminder systems and group education. Incidently, Soumerai and colleagues, who conducted the review on prescribing,[28] also observed that poorly controlled studies were more likely to report significant results than were adequately controlled studies. This highlights the need for rigorous evaluation of dissemination and implementation strategies.

Other behaviours

We have reviewed interventions to improve outpatient referrals, but only found four studies that showed mixed effects.[29] It was difficult to draw any firm conclusions on the basis of the review. In a review of studies of interventions to modify test-ordering behaviour, 15 of 21 studies that targeted a single behavioural factor were successful.[30] However, only two of the 28 studies that targeted more than one behavioural factor were successful.

Grimshaw[29] undertook a review of interventions to improve outpatient referrals. He only identified four studies which showed mixed effects, and stated that it was difficult to draw any firm conclusions on the basis of the review. Solomon and colleagues[30] reviewed 46 studies of interventions to modify test-ordering behaviour. In total, 15 out of 21 studies that targeted a single behavioural factor were successful, whereas two out of 28 studies that targeted more than one behavioural factor were successful.

It seems that multifaceted interventions which target one behavioural factor are more likely to be effective.

Systematic reviews of specific interventions

A total of 16 reviews focused on the effectiveness of specific interventions.

Dissemination of educational materials

Freemantle and colleagues reviewed 11 studies that evaluated the effects of disseminating educational materials (defined as the 'distribution of published or printed recommendations for clinical care, including clinical practice guidelines, audio-visual materials and electronic publications'.[31] The materials may have been delivered personally or by means of personal or mass mailings). None of the studies found statistically significant improvements in practice.

In contrast, the HTA review found 18 studies of dissemination of educational materials, which showed modest but possibly short-lived effects.[16] However, many of the studies were of poor quality and may not portray a true picture of effectiveness.

Educational outreach visits

Thomson O'Brien and colleagues[32] reviewed the effectiveness of educational outreach visits defined as follows:

> The use of a trained person who meets with providers in their practice settings to provide information with the intent of changing the provider's performance. The information given may include feedback on the provider's performance.[32]

They identified 18 studies, mainly targeting prescribing behaviour. The majority of the studies observed statistical improvements in care – especially when social marketing techniques were used – although the effects were small to moderate. Educational outreach was observed to be more effective than audit and feedback in one study. Educational outreach is commonly used in combination with other interventions. The HTA review identified 23 comparisons of multifaceted interventions involving educational outreach.[16] The majority of studies found improvements in the process of care. Compared with the distribution of educational materials alone, eight studies indicated that multifaceted interventions involving educational outreach had modest effects. However, combinations of educational materials and educational outreach appeared to be relatively ineffective. The review findings suggest that educational outreach may produce modest improvements in the process of care, but that this needs to be offset against the resources required to achieve this change.

Local opinion leaders

Thomson O'Brien and colleagues[33] also reviewed the effectiveness of local opinion leaders, defined as 'the use of providers nominated by their colleagues as educationally influential'.

They found improvements in at least one element of the process of care in six of eight studies, although the results were only statistically and clinically significant in two of the trials. In only one trial was there an improvement in patient outcome that was of practical importance. Nevertheless, local opinion leaders were observed to be more effective than audit and feedback in one study. It was concluded that using local opinion leaders resulted in mixed effects. Further research is required before the widespread use of this intervention could be recommended.

Audit and feedback

One review found that feedback was less effective than reminders for reducing the use of diagnostic tests.[34] Balas and colleagues,[35] reviewing 12 evaluations of physician profiling defined as *peer-comparison feedback,* discovered 10 studies that showed statistically significant improvements, but the effects were small. They concluded that peer comparison alone is unlikely to result in substantial quality improvement or cost control, and may be inefficient. In a review by Thomson O'Brien and colleagues,[36] audit and feedback as an intervention was defined as follows:

> Any summary of clinical performance over a specified period of time. Summarised information may include the average number of diagnostic

tests ordered, the average cost per test or per patient, the average number of prescriptions written, the proportion of times a desired clinical action was taken, etc. The summary may also include recommendations for clinical care. The information may be given in a written or verbal format.

A total of 13 studies were found which compared audit and feedback with a no-intervention control group.[36] Eight studies reported statistically significant changes in favour of the experimental group in at least one major outcome measure, but again the effects were small to moderate. The review concluded that 'audit and feedback can be effective in improving performance, in particular for prescribing and test ordering, although the effects are small to moderate'. The widespread use of audit and feedback was not supported by the review.

The HTA review identified 12 comparisons involving the use of audit and feedback as a single intervention, and the results suggested modest effects.[16] Four comparisons of audit and feedback combined with the dissemination of educational materials found modest improvements in care.

Audit and feedback is a commonly used intervention for improving the quality of healthcare. The substantial variation in its effects among studies may be related to differences in context (e.g. whether in primary or secondary care) and to the way in which audit and feedback is conducted (e.g. timing and format of feedback). As with most other interventions, we still know relatively little about what factors constitute the most 'active ingredients' of audit and feedback.

Reminders (manual or computerised)

The effectiveness of computer-based decision support systems (CDSSs) has also been examined. Significant improvements were observed in six of 15 drug-dosing studies, one of five studies on diagnosis, 14 of 19 studies on prevention, 19 of 26 studies on general management of a problem, and four of seven studies on patient outcome.[37] It was concluded that CDSSs may enhance clinical performance for most aspects of care, but *not* for diagnosis.

The HTA review identified 38 comparisons of reminders used as a single intervention, which suggested that their use results in moderate effects.[16] In other studies, the addition of reminders to other interventions increased their effectiveness.

Computerisation

There have been two broader reviews of the effects of computerised systems,[38,39] in one case covering 30 studies on the effects of computers on primary care consultations.[38] It was observed that immunisation, other preventive tasks and some other aspects of performance improved. However, consultation time lengthened, and there was a reduction in patient-initiated social contact. It seems that a range of different computer interventions improve care, including clinician prompts, patient prompts, computer-assisted patient education and computer-assisted treatment planners.[39]

Other interventions

There have also been reviews of other types of intervention – for example, the effects of mass-media campaigns on health services utilisation, where statistical improvements were seen in seven of 17 studies and meta-analysis suggested that campaigns do have an effect.[40] In a systematic review of continuous quality improvement (CQI) programmes, 43 single-site studies (of which 41 studies used an uncontrolled before-and-after design) and 13 multi-site studies (of which 12 studies used a cross-sectional or uncontrolled before-and-after design) were examined.[41] The results from the uncontrolled before-and-after or cross-sectional studies suggested that CQI was effective, whereas none of the randomised studies showed any effect. The predominance of single-site study designs made it difficult to attribute the observed effects to CQI.

Multifaceted interventions

Earlier reviews suggested that combining interventions increased the likelihood of successful implementation, perhaps because of their ability to overcome more than one barrier to change.[42] However, the HTA review found no relationship between the number of component interventions and the effects of multifaceted interventions.[16] Any potential additional benefits associated with multifaceted interventions need to be balanced against their greater costs.

Choosing implementation strategies

Clinical governance leads should ideally have access to a range of proven interventions that can support the implementation of evidence-based practice. However, shopping around for interventions is rather like shopping for clothes – no one style and size suits all shapes and sizes of problem.[43] Most interventions are effective under some circumstances, and none are effective under all circumstances. Just as it is difficult to keep up with changing fashions, clinical governance leads may find tracking the changing evidence base similarly frustrating.

Nevertheless, it is possible to choose a potentially successful strategy in the light of knowledge of the effectiveness of interventions to implement evidence-based practice. Identifying the most important and amenable barriers to change (covered in detail in Chapter 8) represents a key step in the selection of interventions. Table 7.1 lists examples of the rationales that underpin some approaches to changing professional behaviour.[13] However, we emphasise that there is currently little empirical (research-based) evidence to inform the selection of interventions given specific barriers and circumstances. Furthermore, the presence of organisational barriers will require other types of specific interventions.

Resources for implementing evidence-based practice are limited. In some circumstances, the benefits gained from a change in clinical behaviour (e.g. reduced prescribing costs) may be outweighed by the costs of interventions to support that change in behaviour (e.g. educational outreach). Therefore the potential benefits to be gained from targeting a clinical behaviour – whether related to reductions in mortality, morbidity or resource use – need to be considered when selecting an appropriate implementation strategy.[44]

Table 7.1 Examples of rationales for choosing interventions to change professional behaviour

Barrier	Intervention	Rationale
Lack of awareness of research findings	Dissemination of educational materials	Awareness raising
Lack of awareness of need for change	Audit and feedback	Demonstrates need for change or reinforces good practice; also allows use of peer pressure
Cultural barriers to change	Educational outreach; local opinion leaders	Influence of key individuals in social networks
Inability to process all information during consultations	Prompts and reminders	Reduces errors of omission; conditions professionals to practise desired behaviour

Conclusions

Clinical governance requires collaboration between clinicians and managers, who will need access to sources of rigorous evidence. Guidelines and systematic reviews provide the best source of evidence of the effectiveness of healthcare interventions. Reviews of the effectiveness of implementation strategies confirm that the active dissemination and implementation of guidelines is required to ensure that the potential changes in practice occur. There are a variety of evidence-based implementation strategies, each of which is effective under certain conditions.

The choice of strategy should be based on consideration of the following:

* which focused activities should be targeted
* at which specific healthcare professionals they should be targeted
* which perceived barriers to change are to be overcome.

Attention should also be given to likely available resources and the processes needed to manage change.

Practical points

* Evidence-based practice needs to be complemented by evidence-based implementation.
* Passive dissemination on its own does not result in behaviour change.
* No single intervention is effective in all circumstances – there are no 'magic bullets'.
* It is not known whether locally developed guidelines are more effective than national ones – they do need to take account of local circumstances.
* It is more difficult to bring about complex behaviour change.
* Interventions should address perceived barriers to change.

References

1 Royal College of General Practitioners (1985) *Quality in General Practice. Policy Statement 2.* Royal College of General Practitioners, London.

2 Royal College of Radiologists (1995) *Making the Best Use of a Department of Clinical Radiology: guidelines for doctors.* Royal College of Radiologists, London.

3 Secretaries of State for Health and Social Services (1989) *Working for Patients.* HMSO, London.

4 NHS Executive (1996) *Promoting Clinical Effectiveness: a framework for action in and through the NHS.* Department of Health, London.

5 NHS Executive (1996) *Research and Development: towards an evidence-based health service.* Department of Health, London.

6 Johnston G, Crombie IK, Davies HTO, Alder EM and Millard A (2000) Reviewing audit: barriers and facilitating factors for effective clinical audit. *Qual Health Care.* **9**: 23–36.

7 Department of Health (1997) *The New NHS: modern, dependable.* The Stationery Office, London.

8 Eccles M and Grimshaw J (1995) Whither quality assurance? A view from the United Kingdom. *Eur J Gen Pract.* **1**: 8–10.

9 Guyatt G and Rennie D (1993) Users' guides to the medical literature. *JAMA.* **270**: 2096–7.

10 Egger M and Davey Smith G (1998) Bias in location and selection of studies. *BMJ.* **316**: 61–6.

11 Hibble A, Kanka D, Pencheon D and Pooles F (1998) Guidelines in general practice: the new Tower of Babel? *BMJ.* **317**: 862–3.

12 Cluzeau FA, Littlejohns P, Grimshaw JM, Feder G and Moran SE (1999) Development and application of a generic methodology to assess the quality of clinical guidelines. *Int J Qual Health Care.* **11**: 21–8.

13 Grol R (1997) Beliefs and evidence in changing clinical practice. *BMJ.* **315**: 418–21.

14 Alderson P, Bero LA, Grilli R *et al.* (2002) *Cochrane Effective Practice and Organisation of Care Group. The Cochrane Library Issue 4.* Update Software, Oxford.

15 NHS Centre for Reviews and Dissemination (1999) *Getting Evidence into Practice.* University of York, York.

16 Grimshaw JM, Thomas RE, MacLennan G *et al.* (2002) *Effectiveness and Efficiency of Guideline Dissemination and Implementation Strategies.* Health Services Research Unit, University of Aberdeen, Aberdeen.

17 Davis DA, Thomson MA, Oxman AD and Haynes RB (1995) Changing physician performance: a systematic review of the effect of continuing medical education strategies. *JAMA.* **274**: 700–5.

18 Lomas J (1991) Words without action? The production, dissemination and impact of consensus recommendations. *Annu Rev Public Health.* **12**: 41–65.

19 Grilli R and Lomas J (1994) Evaluating the message: the relationship between compliance rate and the subject of a practice guideline. *Med Care.* **32**: 202–13.

20 NHS Centre for Reviews and Disseminations (1994) Implementing clinical practice guidelines. *Effect Health Care.* University of York.

21 Oxman AD, Thomson MA, Davis DA *et al.* (1995) No magic bullets: a systematic review of 102 trials of interventions to improve professional practice. *Can Med Assoc J.* **153**: 1423–31.

22 Wensing M, Van Der Weijden T and Grol R (1998) Implementing guidelines and innovations in general practice: which interventions are effective? *Br J Gen Pract.* **48**: 991–7.

23 Thomas L, Cullum N, McColl E, Rousseau N, Soutter J and Steen N (1999) *Clinical Guidelines in Nursing, Midwifery and Other Professions Allied to Medicine. The Cochrane Library Issue 1.* Update Software, Oxford.

24 Yano EM, Fink A, Hirsch SH, Robbins AS and Rubenstein LV (1995) Helping practices reach primary care goals. Lessons from the literature. *Arch Intern Med.* **155**: 1146–56.

25 Lomas J and Haynes B (1988) A taxonomy and critical review of tested strategies for the application of clinical practice recommendations: from 'official' to 'individual' clinical policy. *Am J Prev Med.* **2**: 77–94.

26 Hulscher M (1998) *Implementing Prevention in General Practice: a study on cardiovascular disease.* University of Nijmegen, Nijmegen.

27 Snell JL and Buck EL (1996) Increasing cancer screening: a meta-analysis. *Prev Med.* **25**: 702–7.

28 Soumerai SB, McLaughlin TJ and Avorn J (1989) Improving drug prescribing in primary care: a critical analysis of the experimental literature. *Milbank Q.* **67**: 268–317.

29 Grimshaw JM (1998) *Evaluation of Four Quality Assurance Initiatives to Improve Outpatient Referrals From General Practice to Hospital.* University of Aberdeen, Aberdeen.

30 Solomon DH, Hashimoto H, Daltroy L and Liang MH (1998) Techniques to improve physicians' use of diagnostic tests. *JAMA.* **280**: 2020–7.

31 Freemantle N, Harvey EL, Wolf F, Grimshaw JM, Grilli R and Bero LA (1999) *Printed Educational Materials: effects on professional practice and health care outcomes. The Cochrane Library Issue 4.* Update Software, Oxford.

32 Thomson O'Brien MA, Oxman AD, Davis DA, Haynes RB, Freemantle N and Harvey EL (2002) *Educational Outreach Visits: effects on professional practice and health care outcomes. The Cochrane Library Issue 4.* Update Software, Oxford.

33 Thomson O'Brien MA, Oxman AD, Haynes RB, Davis DA, Freemantle N and Harvey EL (2002) *Local Opinion Leaders: effects on professional practice and health care outcomes. The Cochrane Library Issue 4.* Update Software, Oxford.

34 Buntinx F, Winkens R, Grol R and Knottnerus JA (1993) Influencing diagnostic and preventative performance in ambulatory care by feedback and reminders. *Fam Pract.* **10**: 219–28.

35 Balas EA, Boren SA, Brown GD, Ewigman BG, Mitchell JA and Perkoff GT (1996) Effect of physician profiling on utilisation. *J Gen Intern Med.* **11**: 584–90.

36 Thomson O'Brien MA, Oxman AD, Davis DA, Haynes RB, Freemantle N and Harvey EL (2002) *Audit and Feedback: effects on professional practice and health care outcomes. The Cochrane Library Issue 4.* Update Software, Oxford.

37 Hunt DL, Haynes RB, Hanna SE et al. (1998) Effects of computer-based clinical decision support systems on physician performance and patient outcomes. *JAMA.* **280**: 1339–46.

38 Sullivan F and Mitchell E (1995) Has general practitioner computing made a difference to patient care? A systematic review of published reports. *BMJ.* **311**: 848–52.

39 Balas EA, Austin SM, Mitchell J, Ewigman BG, Bopp KD and Brown GD (1996) The clinical value of computerised information services. *Arch Fam Med.* **5**: 271–8.

40 Grilli R, Freemantle N, Minozzi S, Domenighetti G and Finer D (1998) *Impact of Mass Media on Health Services Utilisation. The Cochrane Library Issue 3.* Update Software, Oxford.

41 Shortell SM, Bennett CL and Byck GR (1998) Assessing the impact of continuous quality improvement on clinical practice: what will it take to accelerate progress? *Milbank Q.* **76**: 1–37.

42 Cabana MD, Rand CS, Powe NR *et al.* (1999) Why don't physicians follow clinical practice guidelines? A framework for improvement. *JAMA.* **282**: 1458–65.

43 Constantine S and Woodall T (2002) *What Not to Wear.* Weidenfeld and Nicolson, London.

44 Mason J, Freemantle N, Nazareth I, Eccles M, Haines A and Drummond M (2001) When is it cost-effective to change the behaviour of health professionals? *JAMA.* **286**(23): 2988–92.

CHAPTER 8

Quality improvement processes

Richard Baker and Mayur Lakhani

Quality improvement remains the core task of clinical governance. This chapter considers a framework for quality improvement processes for primary care. Although a complete model of clinical governance is not presented, quality improvement is discussed in relation to a more general model illustrated by examples.[1]

Introduction

Four elements must be in place for quality improvement to occur in primary care. The first is the creation of a culture (with its associated systems) that promotes interest in quality and facilitates quality improvement. The second element requires the introduction of systems to identify obstacles to quality and quality improvement. The third element involves developing strategies to overcome the particular obstacles so identified. Fourthly, quality improvement should be targeted at deficiencies in care, and appropriate changes monitored. If improvements do not take place, further action will be required.

Quality systems in organisations

Basic principles

Clinical governance can be regarded as a type of quality system. Almost all moderate-sized commercial or industrial systems will have a quality system, the aim of which is to improve and maintain the quality of performance. The elements of quality systems vary between different organisations, some organisations having more developed systems than others.

The general process of developing a quality system is shown in Figure 8.1.

Typically an organisation will begin by using one quality improvement or implementation method. In the case of the UK National Health Service, that method has been clinical audit. However, one method is never enough because the range of

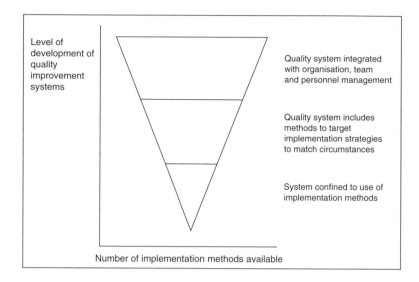

Level of
development of
quality
improvement
systems

Quality system integrated
with organisation, team
and personnel management

Quality system includes
methods to target
implementation strategies
to match circumstances

System confined to use of
implementation methods

Number of implementation methods available

Figure 8.1 The development of quality systems.

problems is always greater than can be solved by any single method alone. Thus as time goes by, a wider range of methods comes into use. At some point it becomes clear that the haphazard use of a variety of methods can lead to much wasted effort and little impact. The various methods have to be brought together and targeted at particular quality problems. One method may be particularly suited to one type of problem, while another method may be more appropriate for other problems. Therefore the next level of development of a quality system is the introduction of a mechanism to identify problems and to target specific methods to be used to overcome them. Quality improvements will take place, but eventually the pace of improvement will slow down again and it will become clear that the final hurdle is the organisational culture itself. If quality is to be guaranteed, the entire organisation needs to be constructed so as to ensure quality performance. This means that the quality system must become integrated with – and virtually indistinguishable from – the general management system.

Getting started in primary care organisations

Dr Silvester had been appointed as the clinical governance lead to the Professional Executive Committee (PEC) of the North Barchester Primary Care Trust. Dr Silvester had been a member of the local Primary Care Audit Group, and had been responsible for involving several local practices in audit. However, she recognised that there would be more to clinical governance than audit alone, but there was very little guidance about how clinical governance should be established or what it would consist of. Her role as clinical governance lead seemed both daunting and ill-defined.

It is possible to assess the level of development of the quality system in a particular primary care organisation, such as a primary care trust, as shown in Figure 8.1. In general, most primary care organisations will be found to be undertaking many discrete activities, but nonetheless are at a relatively early stage of development. Some audit will have been undertaken, as well as a certain amount of education and training. A complaints systems will be operational, and perhaps significant event audit is being encouraged in order to begin to stimulate interest in monitoring and improving patient safety. An appraisal system will be in place, and general practitioners will be making preliminary preparations for revalidation by the General Medical Council. One or two practices will have worked directly with the Primary Care Collaborative, with a particular focus on access or care of people with coronary heart disease. These practices will have gained experience of rapid-cycle data collection, and will be ready to share what they have learned with other local primary care teams. A team from the organisation may even have attended the programme run by the National Clinical Governance Support Unit. Thus a growing number of improvement methods will be in use to varying extents, although as yet they are unlikely to be fully integrated into a comprehensive system that incorporates the four elements, namely culture, identification of obstacles, targeted strategies and monitoring.

The leadership of the primary care organisation must provide direction for the introduction of clinical governance – a particular variety of quality system – to ensure that it gradually develops and becomes effective. The starting point is the creation of an appropriate culture with practical systems of communication and decision making. Quality of care ultimately depends on the performance of individuals. To perform at their best, individuals require the reward of job satisfaction, participation in decision making about their work, support and understanding from the organisation for which they work, and the elimination of obstacles that prevent them from performing to the best of their ability.

Dr Silvester thought about the development of clinical governance in her primary care trust in terms of quality systems in the commercial world. It then became clear that the quality system in her group was at an early stage of development, and that it might take five years or longer to fully implement a reasonable system. She also recognised that it would be of limited value to concentrate her initial effort on merely increasing the range of improvement methods available. Simply promoting more audit and educational activities was not going to be enough. First she needed to gain the support of her Board for a long-term strategy to develop clinical governance in her primary care trust.

The Board had already decided that the clinical governor must be clinically respected and have the confidence of the practitioners within the primary care trust. As Dr Silvester was a well-regarded member of the local audit group, they had decided to appoint her. Of particular importance were her highly developed interpersonal and communications skills. They felt that a confrontational and aggressive approach would be unlikely to succeed at a time when healthcare professionals were feeling particularly threatened and working under conditions of great difficulty and pressure.

The Board had particularly liked the approach recommended in the RCGP document, *Practical Guidance for Clinical Governors*, which suggested treading a course between over-optimism and inactivity in the first year.[2] The Board was keen to ensure that primary healthcare professionals remained committed, and therefore wished to adopt a supportive approach. If the primary care trust had created a clinical governance system that concentrated only on inspection, the consequence would have been loss of motivation among healthcare professionals. Such a bureaucratic approach would have caused healthcare professionals to limit themselves to the bare minimum necessary to comply with clinical governance. In contrast, a culture that valued healthcare professionals and balanced professional autonomy with accountability (without sacrificing the objective of detecting poor performance) would be more likely to lead to successful clinical governance. Dr Silvester and her Board set aside a half-day meeting to discuss these issues and agree their attitude towards clinical governance for the trust.

In our example, the clinical governor and her Board devoted the scarce resource of time to developing their ideas for clinical governance. This would be an appropriate first step for other groups, and having begun to develop ideas about clinical governance among those responsible for leading the group, the next step would be to begin to develop a complementary culture within primary healthcare teams. Culture begins at the top of the organisation, and consequently the support of the Board and the Chief Executive is fundamental. However, more than support is needed. The leaders must be actively engaged in deciding on the culture for clinical governance, and in planning how that culture will be established. They must also recognise that what they do will be more important than what they say in determining culture. Effective communication between the clinical governor and practices is the essential key to developing a culture that is conducive to quality improvement, and the communication must be two-way, open, unimpeded and designed to generate trust. Face-to-face meetings are almost always necessary, but they should be supplemented by comprehensive and rapid written communication. One option would be to visit each primary healthcare team in turn for detailed discussions 'on their turf'. Another option is discussed in the next stage of our example.

Dr Silvester wrote to all primary healthcare teams and identified a clinical governance lead in each of them. She convened a meeting of the leads to discuss the opportunities for and barriers to clinical governance. As a result, the leads agreed on a work plan for the next 12 months. They agreed to invite to their meetings the Primary Care Audit Group general manager and a general practitioner educationalist from the local postgraduate department. The leads identified a framework for developing clinical governance that included plans relevant to individual professionals, primary healthcare teams and the primary care trust as a whole. A pertinent issue for the leads was to establish confidentiality and arrangements for data sharing within

the primary care trust and with the Board. The leads also planned a programme of team visits by clinician peers to develop understanding of each
team's philosophy and its strengths and weaknesses.

The Board recognised that Dr Silvester could not deliver clinical governance alone. Her role was to offer 'leadership in ensuring that the systems are
in place and working', and she should be supported by the primary care
trust in the 'building of alliances to use existing skills and resources to maxi-
mum benefit'.[2] The Board also identified resources as a key issue and decided
to convene a meeting with the health authority to discuss the possibility of
protected time for teams to develop clinical governance. A policy for
clinical governance for non-principals was also to be developed. In addition, the group decided to investigate mechanisms for helping sick
doctors, and to sort out arrangements for an occupational health system
for team members.

Identification of obstacles to change

The organisation of the National Health Service as a whole, the resources available,
and the current environment of continuous change and reform will often present
difficulties to quality improvement in primary care. Although these obstacles
cannot be eliminated, they must be taken into account when anticipating what can
be achieved within a reasonable time. However, it is important not to allow factors
outside the control of the primary care organisation to generate a culture of fatalism.
New ideas for solving old problems can often be generated when staff feel valued,
have some time to think, and are enabled to test out their proposals. Obstacles to
quality improvement may also arise within the primary care organisation itself, or
within primary healthcare teams, or in relation to individual health professionals.
These can often be addressed within the primary care organisation. Box 8.1 lists
examples of such obstacles to quality improvement.

Different approaches are needed to deal with different obstacles.[3] For example,
if morale is low among members of a primary care trust, and they feel unable to
rise to the challenge of quality improvement, providing them with feedback from
audit which shows that their performance is poor will do little to help. It could merely
reinforce their belief that they are powerless to change things, and will depress
morale even further. Instead, they need confident leadership that initiates small
projects which are certain to succeed and as a result will enable self-confidence to
grow.

It follows that a key first and continuing task for clinical governors in primary
care organisations is to identify the obstacles to change that must be faced, becoming attuned to the mood of the primary care trust and the problems confronting the
constituent teams and individuals. A variety of methods may be used to identify
both obstacles to quality improvement and the levers for change that already exist
in the trust. If employed effectively, the levers alone may be sufficient to promote
the quality improvements that are needed. The methods for identifying obstacles
and levers range from informal communication to complex techniques such as
focus groups or surveys of organisational culture.

Box 8.1 Examples of obstacles to quality improvement

Individuals
- Lack of knowledge, skills or time
- Poor personal health
- Not being aware of the need for change
- Not being convinced of the need for change

Teams
- Poor communication about the change
- Conflicting objectives
- Lack of appropriately skilled personnel
- Poor collaboration

Primary care organisations
- Limited resources
- Low morale among members
- Poor communication between healthcare teams
- Lack of leadership
- Low priority given to quality of care

Informal communication is always useful. If you do not understand why implementation of improvement is proving difficult, go and ask the people involved – their answers are often revealing. However, there are some disadvantages to this approach. The respondents may not be representative, and they may be unable to identify the most important obstacles. Formal methods of investigation can allow a more complete description of the obstacles and levers, and can also enable them to be explored in greater depth. The methods cannot be discussed in detail here, but we have included references to full descriptions of how they can be used (*see* Box 8.2). When choosing methods for identifying obstacles and levers, it should be remembered that information is needed about the primary care trust as an organisation, the primary healthcare teams in the trust, and individual professionals. One system for meeting these requirements is shown in Box 8.3.

Box 8.2 Methods of identifying obstacles and levers

Individuals
- Appraisal systems
- Interviews
- Questionnaires

Primary healthcare teams
- Observation of team meetings
- Visits by clinical governance lead to meet with leads of each team
- Reports from team clinical governance leads
- Questionnaires (e.g. the team diagnostic instrument[4])

Primary care group
- Discussion by members of the Board
- Focus groups of members of the primary care group[5]
- Questionnaire about culture[6]
- Questionnaire about teamwork[4]

Box 8.3 A strategy for identifying obstacles and levers in a primary care trust

Individuals
Appraisal system introduced for all health professionals, with appraisal performed by clinical governance lead from neighbouring practices; reports from appraisals collated by the clinical governance lead

Teams
Visit by primary care trust clinical governance lead to each practice to meet with teams; structured interview used during the visits to explore obstacles and levers

Primary care trust
Focus groups convened at intervals – some groups with doctors, some with nurses, some with managers and some with patients

Dr Silvester set up two schemes for identifying obstacles and levers. The first was designed to detect problems in teamwork. She undertook a survey in which members of teams were asked to complete a brief questionnaire on their perceptions of their teamwork. The responses were all dealt with confidentially, but enabled her to identify the strengths and weaknesses of each team.

Nine of the 12 teams appeared to be functioning satisfactorily, but three were in need of help. In one team, the practice manager had been unwell and had had a lot of time off work. At the same time, the practice nurse had retired and a replacement had not been found. Dr Silvester asked the Board to provide emergency support – a senior receptionist from another team was seconded to help with practice management, and a locum practice nurse was found.

In the second team, there were difficulties with communication. Practice meetings were infrequent and members of the team were not involved in making plans. Consequently, the team was failing to respond to the changing demands of healthcare. In response, Dr Silvester arranged for a course organiser from a nearby vocational training scheme to facilitate practice meetings over a period of several months. As a result, the team was able to confront its problems with communication, work together to resolve them, and transform its approach to innovation and development.

The third team was a small inner-city practice facing a heavy workload. The team was overwhelmed and unable to stand back and make plans for long-term development. Day-to-day pressures took precedence over everything else. Dr Silvester discussed this problem with her Board and convinced them of the need for particular support through the provision of a salaried general practitioner and a primary care nurse approved for prescribing. This additional support over the course of the next year enabled the practice to devote more time to planning its future and taking control of its own destiny.

The second scheme was intended to support the individual professionals in the primary care trust. Dr Silvester set in place a personal development appraisal system for all general practitioners and nursing staff. The clinical governance leads in each primary healthcare team were invited to take on the role of appraisal of a team other than their own. The appraisals took place over a period of six months, and as a result every clinician in the primary care trust was able to discuss with a colleague their personal educational needs.

Monitoring performance

Since quality improvement activities cannot be relied upon to be successful, it is important to monitor progress. Clinical audit is the method by which performance can be monitored. All primary healthcare team professionals will now have become familiar with clinical audit, and many detailed descriptions of audit are available.[7] However, since methodological weaknesses have been common in many audits undertaken in recent years, it is worth highlighting a few points.

The first weakness of many audits is the limited use that is made of research evidence. The best current evidence should be used when selecting which aspects of care to assess. Clearly there is little to be gained by expending effort in collecting data when it has not been established which aspects of care are truly important. In audit, review criteria are used to determine what information is needed (*see* Box 8.4 for a definition), and time spent clarifying the evidence to justify each criterion is time well spent. It is possible to reduce the time devoted to searching for evidence by drawing on good-quality systematic reviews, guidelines or audit protocols that have been developed by others.

Box 8.4   Terms used in audit and monitoring

Guidelines
Systematically developed statements to assist practitioner and patient decisions about appropriate healthcare for specific clinical circumstances[8]

Criteria
Systematically developed statements that can be used to assess the appropriateness of specific healthcare decisions, services and outcomes[8]

Audit protocol
A comprehensive set of criteria for a single clinical condition or aspect of organisation[9]

Standard
The percentage of events that should comply with the criterion[7]

Indicator
A measurable element of practice performance for which there is evidence or consensus that it can be used to assess the quality, and thus change in quality, of care provided[9]

The second weakness common to many audits lies in the use of samples. It is not usually necessary to select a sample of patients to be included in an audit, but when large numbers of patients are involved, and when good-quality computerised data are not available, it may be preferable to select a sample. Samples should be representative and of sufficient size to give confidence that the findings do reflect actual practice. Random samples are the safest method of ensuring representative results, and are easy to select. It is also simple to calculate a sample size, although all too often this step is omitted, and consequently the results of the data collection can be misleading. The methods to follow when calculating sample sizes and selecting random samples have been described in detail elsewhere.[7]

The third common problem is failure to complete the cycle. Of course, if performance is already satisfactory, a second data collection would be a waste of time, but usually this happy state of affairs is not the explanation for failure to complete the cycle. If computerised data are not readily available, a second data collection might require extra time and effort, but there is no other way to check that improvements have taken place. Considerable progress is being made in improving information systems in primary care, and primary care organisations can call on external help from experts such as PRIMIS. The new general practitioner contract will accelerate the process of computerisation. However, it is important to follow the principle of collecting the data that you need, rather than collecting the data that are readily available.

A growing number of practices will have experienced rapid-cycle data collection techniques in recent years.[7] This method may offer an alternative to the traditional audit cycle when the topic is relatively discrete and small, incremental changes can be made in clinical or administrative systems (e.g. systems for running a diabetes clinic, or the operation of an appointment system). Good-quality evidence about the effectiveness of rapid-cycle data collection is not yet available, but clinical governors should seek out new methods for quality improvement that might suit the needs and circumstances of their primary healthcare teams.

Conclusion

The principal aim of clinical governance is to improve the quality of care. This requires the creation of an appropriate culture and sense of direction, systems to identify obstacles and levers that influence the success of quality improvement, removal of such obstacles (or overcoming them if they cannot be removed), and monitoring of performance through clinical audit. If these core principles of clinical governance are implemented, primary care teams and organisations should see improvements in the quality of care delivered. Equally, the health professionals within such teams and organisations should find their working lives more enjoyable and fulfilling as a result.

Practical points

- Quality improvement is the core task of clinical governance.
- Experience from commerce and industry is helpful.
- A variety of quality improvement methods is needed.
- A supportive culture is essential.
- Clinical audit, good teamwork and clear communication all play their part.

References

1 Baker R, Lakhani M, Fraser R and Cheater F (1999) A model for clinical governance in primary care groups. *BMJ*. **318**: 779–83.
2 Royal College of General Practitioners (1999) *Practical Guidance on the Implementation of Clinical Governance in England and Wales: a statement from the RCGP*. Royal College of General Practitioners, London.

3   Baker R, Hearnshaw H and Robertson N (1999) *Implementing Change with Clinical Audit.* John Wiley and Sons, Chichester.

4   Pritchard P and Pritchard J (1994) *Teamwork for Primary and Shared Care* (2e). Oxford Medical Publications, Oxford.

5   Krueger RA (1988) *Focus Groups: a practical guide for applied research.* Sage Publications, Newbury Park, CA.

6   Hearnshaw H, Reddish S, Carlyle D, Baker R and Robertson N (1998) Introducing a quality improvement programme to primary healthcare teams. *Qual Health Care.* **7**: 200–8.

7   National Institute for Clinical Excellence (2001) *Principles for Best Practice in Clinical Audit.* Radcliffe Medical Press, Oxford.

8   Field MJ and Lohr KN (eds) (1992) *Guidelines for Clinical Practice: from development to use.* National Academy Press, Washington, DC.

9   Lawrence M and Olesen F for the Equip Working Party on Indicators (1997) Indicators of quality in health care. *Eur J Gen Pract.* **3**: 103–8.

CHAPTER 9

Appropriate use of data: the example of indicators

Richard Thomson

The ultimate criterion for the acceptance of a quality indicator is whether it leads to successful quality improvement projects.

S Jencks[1]

> The quality of primary care has many dimensions. This chapter reviews both the potential and the limitations of quality/performance indicators, with illustrative examples from primary and secondary care. It provides a checklist of questions to ask when the use of indicators is being considered.

Introduction

If clinical governance is to support quality improvement in primary care, the issue of data quality is critical. This is not simply about technical properties, such as validity and reliability. The *quality of data use* is equally important – that is, how data are collected, collated and fed back, who applies the data and the uses to which such data are put.

Although clinical governance incorporates monitoring and accountability, its main emphasis is on continuous quality improvement. There is therefore a challenge in reconciling monitoring, which implies a degree of judgement, with organisation-wide continuous quality improvement. Nowhere is this more evident than in the use of quality/performance indicators.

What is a quality or performance indicator?

An indicator should be a rate, with both a numerator and a denominator. For example, the percentage of patients with diabetes who have had their cardio-vascular risk status reviewed requires as a numerator the number of diabetic patients whose risk factors have been reviewed, and as a denominator the total number of diabetic patients. Further refinement of both the numerator and the denominator allows more valid and reliable data collection, thus ensuring that the data are comparable.

The Joint Commission on Accreditation of Healthcare Organisations (JCAHO) defines an indicator as 'a quantitative measure that can be used to monitor and evaluate the quality of important governance, management, clinical and support functions that affect patient outcomes'. Furthermore, 'an indicator is not a direct measure of quality. Rather, it is a tool that can be used to assess performance and that can direct attention to issues that may require more intense review'.[2] Indicators of performance aim to improve the quality of health services, ultimately resulting in improved patient care and population health.

However, indicators are but flags or screens – they are tools for generating further questions. Examination of an indicator begs the following questions. Why is this rate as it is? Why has it changed? Why does it differ from the rate in another practice or primary care trust area? Such questions can only be answered by further exploration, preferably at a local level. Although indicator data can be collated centrally (and to support comparisons they often need to be), the explanations for a local rate are local – as, more importantly, are the changes needed to improve quality. Thus if primary care trust A has a rate of generic prescribing well below that of other primary care trusts, this merits local investigation, exploring such questions as the following. How does this vary across the primary care trust, from practice to practice, or from GP to GP? Does this reflect a greater level of non-generic prescribing in certain *British National Formulary* chapters or drug types? What are the costs of non-generic prescribing? Where are the largest discrepancies (in terms of both prescription numbers and costs) worthy of exploration? When these questions are answered, yet more questions arise. For example, why are generic prescribing levels low in musculoskeletal and joint diseases? What can we do to change this situation? Is there evidence to support policy or behaviour change? And so on (*see* Box 9.1 for an example).

Box 9.1   Examples of effective use of indicators to improve quality in primary care

Prescribing ratio of inhaled steroids to bronchodilators in Lambeth, Southwark and Lewisham Health Authority
The health authority identified a range of primary care outcome measures, chosen on the basis of relevance to health, patient-centredness, application to broad populations, allowing comparison between providers, and being attributable to primary care interventions. Practices received graphs of their rate compared with the authority mean. One example, namely the prescribing ratio of inhaled steroids to bronchodilators from PACT data, demonstrated variation of approximately fourfold across practices. The data were used as the focus for discussion during pharmaceutical adviser visits. The ratio also contributed to an index that was used to calculate practice prescribing budgets and to identify practices eligible for incentive payments towards more cost-effective prescribing. The local respiratory consultant, who had a special interest in primary care, made contact with practices for which the prescribing ratio suggested that they might have the most to gain from specialist advice or outreach clinics.

Southampton and South-West Hampshire Health Authority primary care indicators
A wide range of indicators was developed to be used in conjunction with information from PACT, the Family Health Services (FHS) Exeter system, the District Child Health system, practice annual reports and the local healthcare purchasing system. A survey revealed that the majority of practices found the indicator set useful. However, the set was primarily used by the health authority's primary care group, and acted as a focus for pharmaceutical adviser and primary care medical adviser practice visits.

As an example, a practice with a high rate of inadequate cervical smears was identified, and this finding was discussed at a subsequent practice visit. This process initiated further training of the practice nurses, which resulted in a marked reduction in the subsequent rate of inadequate smears.

One practice found a relatively low rate of infants being breastfed at six weeks. This led to practice discussion and review, which would not have happened in the absence of comparative data. Thus a previously unidentified issue had been revealed by the indicator.

Source: McColl A, Roderick P and Gabbay J (1997) *Improving Health Outcomes: case studies on how English health authorities use population-based health outcome assessments*. Wessex Institute for Health Research and Development, Southampton.

Types and value of indicators

Indicators have been classified in a number of ways. The commonest classification uses the Donabedian triad of structure, process and outcome, to which can be added access indicators (e.g. waiting times) and activity indicators (e.g. home visit rates). Alternatively, the Department of Health's Performance Assessment Framework initially listed areas (*see* Box 9.2), providing a broad-based approach to assessing the performance of the NHS.[3]

Box 9.2   The NHS Performance Assessment Framework[3]

Area	*Example high-level indicator*
Health improvement	Deaths from all circulatory diseases
Fair access	Adults registered with an NHS dentist
Effective delivery of appropriate care	Cost-effective prescribing
Efficiency	Generic prescribing
Patient/carer experience	First outpatient appointments for which patient did not attend
Health outcomes of NHS care	Emergency admission to hospital for those aged 75 years or over

Most recently, the Department of Health has published performance indicators for primary care organisations (*see* Box 9.3), and the first 'star ratings' for primary care trusts based on these indicators were produced in 2003.[4] These address the full commissioning role of primary care trusts, not only in primary care. As of 2003, the Commission for Health Improvement has taken over the lead role for performance indicators and star ratings following a recommendation in the Kennedy Report of the Bristol Inquiry,[5] and has set up the Office for Information on Health Care Performance. One of its first tasks is to review the indicator sets and their use, including the star-ratings system for primary care trusts.

Box 9.3   Proposed performance indicators for primary care trusts

Area	*Example indicator*
Key targets	Percentage of patients offered an appointment to see a GP within two working days
	Number of patients waiting more than 26 weeks (>21 weeks from end of March 2003) for an outpatient appointment
Access to quality services	Emergency readmissions to hospital following a stroke
	Percentage of patients with HIV appropriately receiving highly active anti-retroviral therapy
Improving health	Death rates from circulatory disease
	Percentage of patients aged 25–64 years screened for cervical cancer
Service provision	Emergency admission rates for asthma and diabetes
	Percentage of resolution of patient complaints within four weeks

For more information, *see* Commission for Health Improvement website.[4]

Quality of care does vary – both between places (geographically) and over time (temporally). Although it may be possible to compare practice rates against published data (e.g. to determine how our primary care team's control of hypertension compares with published audits), the value of the findings is enhanced if there are contemporary data from comparable practice populations. A further potential benefit of comparison lies in the technique of benchmarking (i.e. having identified other teams that appear to be performing better with regard to hypertension control, asking whether we can learn from them). Although this implies being able to review others' rates, it can create concern about the inappropriate use of such comparisons. This worry can be overcome either by identifying voluntary benchmark partners (as hospitals do in the Performance Benchmarking Network), or through a system that uses anonymised data but which identifies and disseminates good practice.

Technical characteristics of indicators

McColl and colleagues[6] have stated that performance indicators for routine use by primary care should:

- be attributable to healthcare
- be sensitive to change
- be based on reliable and valid information
- be precisely defined
- reflect important clinical areas
- include a variety of dimensions of care.

To this one could add that they should be measurable (quantifiable) and timely and, for indicators reflecting clinical treatment, evidence based. Unfortunately, an indicator that fully meets all of these criteria does not exist. Instead, one has to consider the degree to which indicators meet these criteria, alongside other features. For example, an indicator could have good technical characteristics, but vary little from place to place, or reflect an area where change is difficult. All other things being equal, these factors may limit its value compared with other, less technically sound indicators. Furthermore, the use to which indicators will be put will also influence the relative importance of such criteria.

McColl and colleagues[6] describe an approach for linking performance indicators to appropriate evidence-based interventions by:

- identifying interventions for which primary care has a key responsibility and which are of proven value, and
- estimating the potential burden of preventable deaths if the intervention is appropriately applied.

For example, influenza vaccination of all eligible patients aged over 65 years in a population of 100 000 could prevent 146 deaths and 273 influenza episodes annually. If uptake was only 30%, 102 deaths and 191 influenza episodes could be prevented by full coverage. A primary care trust could review comparative data on the percentage of the population vaccinated, and could feed the data back to primary care teams. This would enable them to compare their rate with others, and to monitor change in uptake over time. A primary care trust might then need to decide whether to address this area. What is the current local rate of uptake? How would the effort of creating change compare with, for example, increasing the use of aspirin after myocardial infarction or transient ischaemic attack? How best could the change be supported? (e.g. by targeting individual teams, incorporating it in continuing professional developmental programmes, local media campaigns, etc.) (*see* Chapter 7).

Campbell and colleagues[7] have developed an alternative approach which combines appraisal of the literature with structured expert opinion to develop relevant indicators (review criteria). A long list of potential indicators, garnered from review and appraisal of both the literature and guidelines in the areas of asthma, angina and diabetes, was considered by a consensus panel of experts. Two rounds of anonymous rating, for both necessity and appropriateness, with feedback to panellists of aggregate scores between rounds, were followed by face-to-face discussion. The emerging consensus was thus informed by the combined panel ratings and their variance. 'Strong scientific evidence' was present for only 26% of the potential indicators, which were rated as necessary aspects of care. Thus if the development of indicators was based on randomised controlled trial evidence alone, a very limited number would have been generated, excluding many key elements of 'good' primary care practice. Many primary care interventions, such as the use of practice diabetic registers, could never be the subject of a randomised controlled trial.

The methods of McColl and Campbell offer potentially complementary approaches to developing relevant indicators for use in primary care. These are more likely to gain the approval of the professions, mainly because the development processes are seen as valid.

Data quality and accessibility

The use of indicators is highly dependent on the quality of the underlying data source – data should be both complete and accurate. Thus the rate of aspirin treatment in angina, based on disease-coded data, would require denominator data to be complete (i.e. all patients with angina have a diagnostic coding) and accurate (i.e. patients coded as having angina really do have it). Furthermore, production of these data from the information system should be straightforward.

Attribution to healthcare

Indicators may vary in their degree of attribution to primary care, and thus in their relevance for primary care quality improvement. For example, the uptake of cervical screening is highly attributable to primary care (although of course patients may refuse to be screened), whereas the rate of emergency psychiatric admissions (an indicator proposed as a measure of the outcome of healthcare in the consultation preceding the NHS Performance Assessment Framework[3]) will depend partly on primary care, but also on the relevant social services provision and other factors.

Sensitivity to change

An indicator reflecting clinical practice should be sensitive to change. For example, decreasing the mortality from acute myocardial infarction is the goal of secondary prevention with aspirin, but monitoring this at a practice level using mortality is inappropriate. The numbers involved are too small, and monitoring changes in mortality will be insensitive to changes in the quality of care (*see* Box 9.4).

Box 9.4 The capacity to detect real differences in quality

Mant and Hicks[8] considered the situation of a hospital that admitted 450 patients per year to its coronary care unit with a diagnosis of myocardial infarction. The aim was to monitor the quality of care given over time. In order to detect a significant improvement in *outcome* (a reduction in mortality from 30% to 29%) with confidence, 73 years of data collection would be needed. In contrast, to detect with confidence a significant improvement in a *process* of care (percentage of patients prescribed thrombolytic therapy), which would lead to an equivalent reduction in mortality from 30% to 29%, only four months of data collection would be required. The same issue is highlighted in comparisons between hospitals. The authors concluded that 'even with data aggregated over three years, with a perfect severity adjustment system and identical case ascertainment and definition, disease-specific mortality rates are an insensitive tool to compare the quality of care between hospitals'.

Reliable, valid and comprehensive

An indicator should measure what it seeks to measure (validity) and do so consistently (reliability). Validity is a complex concept. Suffice it to say that a measure is valid if:

- it is a potential marker for quality of primary care (face validity or relevance) and
- it measures what it purports to measure (e.g. a Read-coded stroke reflects a gold standard diagnosis of stroke).

An indicator is reliable if it is collected consistently in different places by different people at different times. This is highly dependent on clear definitions and repeatable methods of data collection.

Campbell and colleagues undertook a national survey of potential indicators of primary care quality and identified 240 such indicators.[9] These were then tested for face validity in a survey of managers and GPs. Only 36 of the indicators scored highly for validity, and the final list included no indicators for effective communication, care of acute illness, health outcomes or patient evaluation. Prescribing and gatekeeper indicators consistently received low validity ratings.

This is important in view of the fact that the quality of primary care has so many dimensions. Concentrating on the measurable may exclude important domains of quality. And even a set of indicators – such as the proposed primary care clinical effectiveness indicators – cannot at present cover all of the relevant domains. Indicators relevant to important dimensions, such as advocacy and consultation skills, would be very difficult to incorporate into any package. Nonetheless, a set of indicators should at least seek to address a range of relevant areas. The difficulty of this, in the light of Campbell's study, is clear.

How can indicator data support quality of care?

Internal or external use?

Anyone who is using or interpreting indicators to improve quality of care needs to be aware of their limitations as well as their potential. This chapter includes examples from various sources, not all of them from primary care or from the UK. Nonetheless, they illustrate the key issues.

A fundamental decision is whether indicators will be used to make (external) judgements or to stimulate further investigation and quality improvement activity (from within), and indeed whether these different uses are compatible. Indicators could be used to make judgements. For example, is primary care team A better than team B? Is Dr Smith's prescribing of higher quality than Dr Jones's? This use is substantively different to feedback of anonymised comparative data to teams in order to support their own clinical audit or service development. Both approaches might be used in concert, but this is not without problems.[10-13] This whole issue has become even more pertinent with proposals that the new GP contract will incorporate incentives in the form of quality payments that are predominantly based on measures/indicators related to chronic disease management.[14]

The reasons why external judgement of performance indicators may be inappropriate include the following:

- quality of primary care data
- choice of measure
- perverse incentives
- case-mix and context
- ability to distinguish
- chance.

Quality of primary care data

Although many practices are now computerised, and most use computers for prescribing (particularly repeat prescribing), computerised data are still limited. Few practices record diagnostic data, and where they do, their completeness and accuracy vary. This problem of missing and inaccurate data has significant implications for both the selection and interpretation of indicators.

Even where data are more complete and accurate, such as PACT data, problems remain.[15] PACT data cannot be linked either to diagnoses or to individual patients to compare the appropriateness of prescribing at a diagnostic level. Equally, PACT data cannot be used to compare age- and gender-corrected prescribing adequately.

Developments in general practice computing and decision-support technology may make future clinical data both more accessible and more complete for comparative analysis. For example, the PRODIGY system provides computerised guidelines with the potential to capture data that are relevant to clinical decisions on specific patients.

McColl and colleagues assessed the capacity of primary care computer systems to provide data for 26 of their evidence-based process indicators, and found that only eight could be derived in all of the 18 practices, and only three practices could derive data for all 26 indicators.[16]

Choice of measure

Judgements imply ranking of practices. Not all of the available measures might be used, and the indicators that are used will exclude important domains of quality (*see* above). Furthermore, the relative ranking of an organisation on the basis of performance indicators depends critically on which indicators are used (*see* Box 9.5).

Box 9.5 Choice of indicator in coronary artery bypass surgery

Hartz and Kuhn[17] used a range of outcome measures and data sources (both clinical and administrative) from 17 US hospitals (with a total of 2687 coronary artery bypass surgery patients) to compare risk-adjusted rates. The correlations between adjusted hospital rankings, derived from either the clinical or the administrative databases, were not statistically significant for mortality, major complications, or indeed for any complication. Although there was a reasonable correlation between risk-adjusted hospital rankings using the clinical database for mortality and major complications, the correlation between major complications and any complication was negative. These results suggested not only that assessing the quality of care by the use of administrative data may not be adequate but also, importantly, that quality assessment using clinical data may depend substantially on the outcome measure used. Thus a hospital with a high ranking on the basis of one outcome measure may have a low ranking if other measures are used.

Perverse incentives

Indicator-based judgements may create perverse incentives. Participants will seek to do well on the chosen indicators. For example, the publicly available Patient's Charter indicators included the percentage of patients seen in Accident and Emergency units within five minutes. This sought to reflect the importance of immediacy of care to patients, and potentially to patient outcome. However, Accident and Emergency departments appointed or redeployed 'triage' nurses, thereby producing improvements in the indicator, but not necessarily better care. Effective triage takes more than five minutes, so the response in many centres was simply to create the perjoratively titled 'hello nurse' – there to greet but not to treat. Comparisons of performance against this indicator showed no correlation between the rating awarded and either the use of full triage or the length of triage.[18]

Some of the originally proposed primary care effectiveness indicators could have similarly perverse effects. An indicator on district nurse visits to the over-75s might lead to an inappropriate reduction in visits to the under-75s. This has been dropped from the NHS Performance Assessment Framework.[3] The ratio of inhaled corticosteroids and cromoglycate to inhaled bronchodilators could be increased by the indiscriminate prescription of steroid inhalers, with little improvement in patient care, and at increased cost. Comparing the rates of complaints might dissuade practices from seeking patient views. A practice with more complaints may have better systems for seeking patient views, rather than poorer care.

Case-mix and context

Indicators are dependent on many factors beyond just the quality of care. Outcome measures in particular depend not only on the structures and processes of care, but also on patient characteristics such as age, sex, comorbidity and socio-economic status. Thus it may be appropriate for a practice based in an area of socio-economic deprivation to have higher prescribing or admission rates.

An inadequate understanding of this can lead to quite erroneous judgements, which cannot be fully ameliorated by adjusting for case-mix (i.e. making allowances for the particular mix of population and conditions). It is not simply a matter of adjusting for extraneous factors to isolate variations that might be due to differences in quality of care. Even with a high-quality, validated, case-mix adjustment system, problems can arise (*see* Box 9.6). Furthermore, the method of adjustment can affect ranking (*see* Box 9.7). Once again, judgements need to be made with extreme caution. This has been explored with reference to the use of risk adjustment methods to support better decisions on capitation-based funding, and it was concluded that in the UK primary care setting the use of risk adjustment when monitoring performance should be explored further.[19]

Box 9.6   The New York State CABG register

The New York State coronary artery bypass graft (CABG) register provides an example of a potential problem. This is a system of comparative, surgeon-specific, risk-adjusted CABG mortality rates which are made publicly available. The system uses a well-developed risk-adjustment process and good clinical data extracted by trained data collectors, with systems of data audit and quality control.[20–22]

Following its introduction, it was noted that low-volume surgeons (those performing fewer operations) had consistently higher risk-adjusted mortality rates. Between 1989 and 1992, a total of 27 low-volume surgeons (with a combined risk-adjusted mortality rate of 11.9%, compared with a statewide average of 3.1%) stopped performing CABG operations in New York State. In one hospital the cardiac surgery programme had to be suspended until a new chief could be recruited, and some hospitals reportedly assigned patients to selected surgeons.[21,22]

A case study from St Peter's Hospital, Albany, New York showed how such data might be used beneficially.[23] This hospital had a high risk-adjusted mortality rate, and decided to investigate further. It was found that this was due not to higher-than-expected mortality among the low-risk patients, but to high rates of mortality among emergency cases. It was felt that not enough time was devoted to stabilising patients. Following a restructuring of care, marked improvements were seen in the mortality rates in this subgroup, from a pre-intervention rate of 11 deaths among 42 emergencies in 1992, to a post-intervention period when none out of 52 emergencies died. This was achieved without the avoidance of high-risk patients, and demonstrates the importance of local audit, and subsequent change, in response to indicator data. It also shows that risk-adjusted data need careful interpretation. Overall, this hospital had a lower-risk population of patients, but their higher apparent mortality was actually due to a problem with high-risk patients.

It is also reported that case-mix-adjusted mortality, in the state as a whole, decreased over time following the introduction of the register, from 4.2% in 1989 to 2.7% in 1991.[24] However, a further analysis of the same data revealed that the recording rate for risk modifiers such as renal failure, congestive heart failure and unstable angina rose markedly over the same period.[25] For example, the rate of recorded renal failure increased from 0.4% to 2.8%, and the rate of chronic obstructive airways disease increased from 6.9% to 17.4%. This may reflect better recording of comorbidity data as the system matured, but the size of the change suggests another explanation – that of gaming (i.e. clinicians recording comorbidities as well). There is a perverse incentive for clinicians to record comorbidities in order to 'upstage' the patient's risk and thereby show mortality rates in a better light.

Box 9.7   Effect of risk-adjustment methods on ranking

Iezzoni and colleagues used 14 different severity adjustment methods when comparing mortality rates for pneumonia in 105 hospitals.[26] Whereas all of the methods produced agreement on relative hospital performance more often than would be expected by chance, 30 hospitals were classified as outliers by one or more methods. The choice of method could therefore have an important effect on the perceived performance of hospitals.

Ability to distinguish

We have already seen the difficulties that arise in demonstrating significant change in the quality of care where indicators cover only small numbers (*see* Box 9.4). This problem also impinges on the capacity to distinguish *between* providers on the basis of differences in indicators. Thus there may be a real difference in quality of care but an inability to demonstrate it (i.e. the indicators chosen may not be sensitive enough).

The play of chance

Given the nature of health and healthcare, chance itself may lead to apparent differences between primary care teams or individual practitioners. This may lead to either false denigration (i.e. things appear worse than they are in reality) or false reassurance (i.e. things appear better than they are in reality).

Conclusions and lessons for primary care

The use of data to support clinical governance and quality improvement has been discussed with specific reference to quality or performance indicators. These have been the focus of considerably more debate since the publication of *A First-Class Service*[27] and *The NHS Performance Assessment Framework*,[3] against a background of public concern following the Bristol case. This chapter has reviewed both the potential and the limitations of the use of such data in primary care. There are lessons to learn for primary care trusts – from past experience in other sectors and other countries (particularly in secondary care). Equally, there is a growing awareness that these issues are generic, regardless of the sector in which indicators are used.

Box 9.8 lists a series of questions and issues that primary care trusts and primary care professionals with a role in clinical governance might ask themselves when considering the use of data and indicators. Box 9.9 lists sources of useful information and further reading.

Box 9.8 Relevant questions to ask of the use of data and indicators in primary care

- What are we seeking to achieve in the use of these data?
- Who will use the data? Will it be publicly available?
- Will the data be used to make judgements or to support clinical audit?
- Who will interpret the data?
- If judgements are to be made, how can we avoid or minimise the potential adverse effects of this approach?
- Will the data be anonymised or will primary care teams be identifiable?
- Where will the data come from? Is it readily accessible?
- What is the quality of the data source?
- Will we derive or collect our own data or use other readily available sources?
- Are the data items, and indicators derived from them, valid, reliable and sensitive to change?
- Are the definitions of data items clear and precisely defined?
- Do they reflect an important area of quality of care?
- Is this attributable to primary care?
- Is there evidence of important variation?
- Is the range of indicators reflective of the range of domains of quality in primary care?

- Are they based on evidence of effectiveness or consensus on good practice?
- Is there opportunity to create change?
- How will we engage local primary care teams and practitioners in the process?
- How will we support teams in the better use of such data?

Box 9.9   Sources of useful information and further reading

Websites
NHS Clinical Governance Support Team
www.cgsupport.org
CHI 'Rating the NHS'
www.chi.nhs.uk/eng/ratings/index.shtml
Scottish Clinical Indicators Support Team
www.show.scot.nhs.uk/indicators
National Primary Care Research and Development Centre (includes guidance on clinical governance and primary care indicators)
www.npcrdc.man.ac.uk/
Clinical Governance Research and Development Unit
www.le.ac.uk/cgrdu
UK Quality Indicator Project (a UK-based project that provides anonymised comparative feedback primarily for secondary and long-term care)
www.newcastle.ac.uk/qip/
AHCPR Indicators CONQUEST database (a database of potential indicators with increasing links to the evidence base)
www.ahcpr.gov/qual/conquest.htm
The NHS Performance Ratings and Indicators 2002
www.doh.gov.uk/performanceratings/2002
and
www.doh.gov.uk/performanceratings/2003

Further reading
- Marshall M, Campbell S, Harker J and Roland M (2002) *Quality Indicators for General Practice: a practical guide for health care professionals and managers.* RSM Publishing, London.
- Roland BO and Baker R (1999) *Handbook – Clinical Governance: a practical guide for primary care teams.* University of Manchester, Manchester.
- Lally J and Thomson RG (1999) Is indicator use for quality improvement and performance measurement compatible? In: H Davies, M Tavakoli, M Malek and A Neilson (eds) *Managing Quality: strategic issues in healthcare management.* Ashgate Publishing, Aldershot.
- Crombie IK and Davies HTO (1998) Beyond health outcomes: the advantages of measuring process. *J Eval Clin Pract.* **4**: 31–8.

Practical points

- A quality or performance indicator should be a rate, with both a numerator and a denominator.
- As far as possible indicators should be attributable to healthcare, precisely defined, based on complete, accurate, valid and reliable data, reflect important and evidence-based aspects of care, and be sensitive to change.
- Such indicators are not available for a number of important dimensions of good-quality primary care.
- Indicators may be used for external judgement and/or for internal quality improvement of an organisation, but different uses may have very different effects.
- Primary care can learn from experience in other sectors (particularly secondary care) and in other countries (particularly the USA).

References

1 Jencks SF (1994) HCFA's Health Care Quality Improvement Program and the Co-operative Cardiovascular Project. *Ann Thorac Surg.* **58**: 1858–62.
2 Joint Commission on Accreditation of Health Care Organisations (1990) *Primer on Indicator Development and Application.* Joint Commission on Accreditation of Health Care Organisations, Chicago.
3 Department of Health (1999) *The NHS Performance Assessment Framework.* Department of Health, London.
4 CHI website: www.chi.nhs.uk/eng/ratings/index.shtml
5 Public Inquiry (2001) *The Report of the Public Inquiry into Children's Heart Surgery at the Bristol Royal Infirmary 1984-95: learning from Bristol.* The Stationery Office, London.
6 McColl A, Roderick P, Gabbay J, Smith H and Moore M (1998) Performance indicators for primary care groups: an evidence-based approach. *BMJ.* **317**: 1354–60.
7 Campbell SM, Roland MO, Shekelle PG, Cantrill JA, Buetow SA and Cragg DK (1998) Development of review criteria for assessing the quality of management of stable angina, adult asthma, and non-insulin-dependent diabetes mellitus in general practice. *Qual Health Care.* **8**: 6–15.
8 Mant J and Hicks N (1995) Detecting differences in quality of care: the sensitivity of measures of process and outcome in treating acute myocardial infarction. *BMJ.* **311**: 793–6.
9 Campbell SM, Roland MO, Quayle JA, Shekelle PG and Buetow S (1999) Quality indicators for general practice: which ones can general practitioners and health authority managers agree are important and how useful are they? *J Public Health Med.* **20**: 414–21.
10 Davies HTO and Lampel J (1998) Trust in performance indicators? *Qual Health Care.* **7**: 159–62.
11 Crombie IK and Davies HTO (1998) Beyond health outcomes: the advantages of measuring process. *J Eval Clin Pract.* **4**: 31–8.
12 McKee M and Hunter D (1995) Mortality league tables: do they inform or mislead? *Qual Health Care.* **4**: 5–12.

13 Thomson R and Lally J (1998) Clinical indicators: do we know what we're doing? *Qual Health Care.* **7**: 122–3.

14 Marshall M and Roland M (2000) The new contract: renaissance or requiem for general practice? *Br J Gen Pract.* **52**: 531–2.

15 Majeed A, Evans N and Head P (1997) What can PACT tell us about prescribing in general practice? *BMJ.* **315**: 1515–19.

16 McColl A, Roderick P, Smith H *et al.* (2000) Clinical governance in primary care groups: the feasibility of deriving evidence-based performance indicators. *Qual Health Care.* **9**: 90–7.

17 Hartz AJ and Kuhn EM (1994) Comparing hospitals that perform coronary artery bypass surgery: the effect of outcome measures and data sources. *Am J Public Health.* **84**: 1609–14.

18 Edhouse JA and Wardrope J (1996) Do the national performance tables really indicate the performance of an Accident and Emergency department? *J Accid Emerg Med.* **13**: 123–6.

19 Majeed A, Bindman AB and Winer JP (2001) Use of risk adjustment in setting budgets and measuring performance in primary care. II. Advantages, disadvantages and practicalities. *BMJ.* **323**: 607–10.

20 Hannan EL, Kumar D, Racz M, Siu AL and Chassin MR (1994) New York State's cardiac surgery reporting system: four years later. *Ann Thorac Surg.* **58**: 1852–7.

21 Hannan EL, Siu AL, Kumar D, Kilburn H and Chassin MR (1995) The decline in coronary artery bypass graft surgery mortality in New York State. *JAMA.* **273**: 209–13.

22 Chassin MR, Hannan EL and DeBuono BA (1996) Benefits and hazards of reporting medical outcomes publicly. *NEJM.* **334**: 394–8.

23 Dziuban SW, McIlduff JB, Miller SJ and Dal Col RH (1994) How a New York cardiac surgery program uses outcomes data. *Ann Thorac Surg.* **58**: 1871–6.

24 Hannan EL, Kilburn HJ, Racz M, Shields E and Chassin MR (1994) Improving the outcomes of coronary artery bypass surgery in New York State. *JAMA.* **271**: 761–6.

25 Green J and Wintfeld N (1995) Assessing New York State's approach. *NEJM.* **332**: 1229–32.

26 Iezzoni LI, Schwartz M, Ash AS, Hughes JS, Daley J and Mackiernan YD (1996) Severity measurement methods and judging hospital death rates for pneumonia. *Med Care.* **34**: 11–28.

27 Department of Health (1998) *A First-Class Service: quality in the NHS.* Department of Health, London.

CHAPTER 10

Managing information

Alan Gillies and Beverley Ellis

This chapter explores the provision of good data for monitoring the quality of primary care. Three issues need to be addressed, namely the kit (IT infrastructure), the way it is used, and the capability of the people who are using it.

Introduction

Clinical governance and information management are inextricably linked. And information is not simply what gets recorded in electronic or paper-based health records. In its broadest sense, information is a crucial part of the clinical process – as can be seen, for example, from the conclusions of the Bristol Inquiry.

For if inadequate quality of care was the symptom in the Bristol case, then arguably inadequate management of information was the root cause that affected each critical stage in the process of care.

- Inadequate information was provided for the parents of patients.
- There were inadequate mechanisms for communicating concerns (i.e. the whistleblowers found that there was no system for facilitating disclosure).
- There was insufficient information to benchmark performance. There were inadequate systems in place to highlight the problems, and even at the point when it was recognised that something was wrong, it was not possible to compare success rates at Bristol with those elsewhere.

Interestingly, these same issues have arisen in relation to adverse healthcare events in other parts of the world.[1]

The Chief Medical Officer, Sir Liam Donaldson, highlighted the problems that whistleblowers experience:

> In the past the health service whistleblower would blow but no one would hear or listen. The dog couldn't bark, so even though the dog was running in their midst to the tune of the silent whistle, no one acknowledged its presence. The problem was there but it wasn't recognised. If it was pointed out, it wasn't acknowledged.[2]

The need to protect whistleblowers has now been recognised by the 1999 Public Disclosure Act.[3] Under the Act and associated guidance, all NHS trusts and health authorities are expected to:

- designate a senior manager to deal with employees' concerns and to protect whistleblowers
- have in place local policies and procedures and set out minimum requirements
- provide guidance to all staff so that they know how to speak up against mal-practice
- provide whistleblowers with adequate protection against victimisation
- prohibit 'gagging' clauses in contracts of employment.

However, Donaldson went on to say that the need is not to make whistleblowing easier, but rather to establish cultures and systems within organisations that remove the need for whistleblowing, through systematic monitoring of clinical care. This chapter explores the provision of good surveillance data in primary care.

Historical developments

Clinical audit was introduced in the 1989 White Paper *Working for Patients*,[4] and was defined at the time as:

> The systematic critical analysis of the quality of medical care, including the procedures used for the diagnosis and treatment, the use of resources and the resulting outcome and quality of life for the patient.[5]

This limited scope can be compared with the more all-embracing definition that is clinical governance.[6] There were also a number of aspects of the way in which clinical audit was carried out that precluded it from providing the safeguards which might have prevented the events at Bristol.

- Clinical audit did not of itself question clinical practice. In general, clinical audit examined process and procedure, and did not question the professional attributes of individual clinicians. The emphasis was on the audit of cohorts of patients, rather than on the care of individuals.
- Clinical audit was applied to topics chosen by clinicians, and there was little involvement of managers or patients.[7] Clinical governance is intended to be more comprehensive and systematic. It covers all aspects of care, and the Commission for Health Improvement monitors the organisations and their systems.
- Clinical audit was regarded as an 'add-on', and was based on data specifically compiled for the specific audit. It was rarely possible to use routinely collected data.

As early as 1992, the NHS Information Management and Technology (IM&T) strategy stated that:

> Subject to safeguards to maintain the confidentiality of personal health information, data will be obtained from systems used by healthcare

professionals in their day-to-day work. There should be little need for different systems to capture information specifically for management purposes.[8]

In the event, the infrastructure did not provide the required information directly, and each audit required its own data collection – usually by trawling through paper records to provide data for entry into a personal computer for analysis. Indeed, the statement that it was expected that by the year 2000 all large acute hospitals would have 'a set of integrated systems' now appears rather naive. Nevertheless, systems are now being implemented that allow audits to be carried out directly on clinical data. This means that clinical audit can be both routine and integrated into operational patient care for the first time. In order to achieve this, we need not only appropriate information systems but also appropriate working practices and human capability.

Implementing effective information systems

Although the focus here is on primary care, the same principles apply to all areas of care. Any effective information system has three essential elements:

1 *infrastructure* – this includes the computer hardware, infrastructure (including networks) and software systems
2 *working processes* – this includes the way in which data are entered into the system to ensure that they can be retrieved and analysed
3 *people* – all staff must be capable of undertaking what they need to do.

The Department of Health has set infrastructure standards for clinical systems, namely the rules for the accreditation of GP systems. In the past these were quite permissive in their definitions and requirements, but there is now a movement towards greater prescription to encourage easy communication between systems.[9] In practice, this means that local primary care trusts will have much less control over and choice of IT infrastructure. However, they will have the job of making sure that the internal processes and human capacity are adequate to deliver the required information for clinical governance and other management functions.

In the past, computerisation in primary care has been largely unplanned. Practices have been free to select the type and timing of computer installation, and have geared up to use the system at their own pace. A more systematic approach is now possible, combining two well-tried management techniques:

• a *maturity model* to define the processes needed to produce effective information
• a *training needs model* to ensure that staff are equipped to operate those processes.

A maturity model

The idea of a maturity model is based on the capability maturity model (CMM) developed by the Software Engineering Institute of Carnegie Mellon University. Their CMM was developed for the US Department of Defence, and defined a five-level framework for how an organisation matures its software processes from *ad hoc* chaotic processes to mature disciplined software processes.[10] The key characteristics of the CMM that can be used in primary care are definition of the characteristics of key stages of maturity, definition of the key actions required to move from one stage to the next, and use of a questionnaire survey to facilitate the analysis of current maturity.

Thus the General Practice Information Maturity Model (GPIMM) describes information management maturity levels for primary care. In simple terms it is a snapshot of how well developed the organisation's information processes are. It is similarly based on five maturity levels, with an additional zero level for non-computerised practices. The maturity levels of the GPIMM are summarised in Table 10.1. Even after more than ten years of computerisation, many practices still operate at the lower levels of the model. This is a significant barrier to effective clinical governance. The reality is that unless practices have procedures at level 4 or above, they will be unable to deliver useful information for clinical governance from their systems.

Table 10.1 Levels of the General Practice Information Maturity Model

Level	Designation	Summary description
0	Paper based	The practice has no computer system
1	Computerised	The practice has a computer system, but it is only used by the practice staff
2	Computerised PHCT	The practice has a computer system, and both the practice staff and the primary healthcare team (PHCT), including the doctors, use it
3	Coded	The system makes limited use of Read codes
4	Bespoke	The system is tailored to the needs of the practice through agreed coding policies and the use of clinical protocols
5	Paperless	The practice is completely paperless, except where paper records are a legal requirement

The GPIMM framework provides a means for practices to develop further to improve their use of their systems. It should be noted that development will not usually require investment in new systems, but rather it will involve extracting greater benefit from existing ones.

- At level 0, the practice is entirely based on paper records. According to official statistics, by 1998 this level represented less than 2% of practices.
- At level 1, the computer has arrived. Typically it is used in a limited way by administrative staff to assist in income generation by monitoring items that attract practice reimbursement. Crucially, it is not used by clinicians in the consultation.
- At level 2, the computer is used by clinicians in a limited way. The practice has started to use the computer to store clinical information. However, that information is stored as free text, so the system is merely an electronic notepad. None of the potential advantages can be realised while information is stored in this way.

- At level 3, the practice has started to code clinical information. Coding will be limited, and the practice may not yet have fully formed policies to ensure that coding is consistent. Some benefits may be realised, but much work remains to be done.
- At level 4, coding is well established, as are policies to ensure that codes are consistent and compatible with primary care trust standards, to allow the practice to take part in local initiatives with other practices. At this stage the system starts to deliver benefits that outweigh the effort required to make it work, and it can support clinical governance as a routine activity.
- At level 5, the practice is effectively operating in electronic fashion. Future developments are in the areas of continuous improvement and links with other agencies.

The GPIMM framework allows the primary care trust to survey practices and to define information strategies for each of them, providing a structured improvement process to get practices to the required level. The maturity level may be assessed by means of a computerised questionnaire that covers five areas:

1 *computerisation* – this is simply a filter to identify those practices that remain paper based
2 *personnel usage* – this section examines the impact of the system on the practice; any system's potential usefulness is severely limited if it is only used by practice staff
3 *coding* – this section is crucial, as it considers not only the extent of coding but also the quality of coding, by examining the policies and internal consultation that underpin coding practice
4 *system usage* – this section is concerned with the impact that the system has on the working methods of the practice; it measures the extent to which the system works for the practice, not the other way around
5 *electronic patient records* – this section reviews how far the electronic patient record is realised both inside and outside the practice.

The GPIMM is a model designed for use by primary care trusts as a computerised tool to survey practice computerisation (*see* Figure 10.1). (Further information can be obtained from bsellis@uclan.ac.uk).

The tool also provides a structured improvement route and a progress report (*see* Figure 10.2).

A training needs model

In order to deliver the process improvement defined by the GPIMM, it is also necessary to ensure that the personnel involved have the required skills. For each level of the GPIMM, required levels of competency have been defined for the key players in primary care, namely GPs, nurses, managers and administrators. Competencies are defined at one of five levels (from novice through to expert), building on the classification developed by Dreyfus and Dreyfus.[11] Thus a training needs matrix may be defined for each GPIMM level (*see* Table 10.2).

The skills of the staff may then be audited against the skills required for the current or target GPIMM level, and training can be tailored to ensure that the

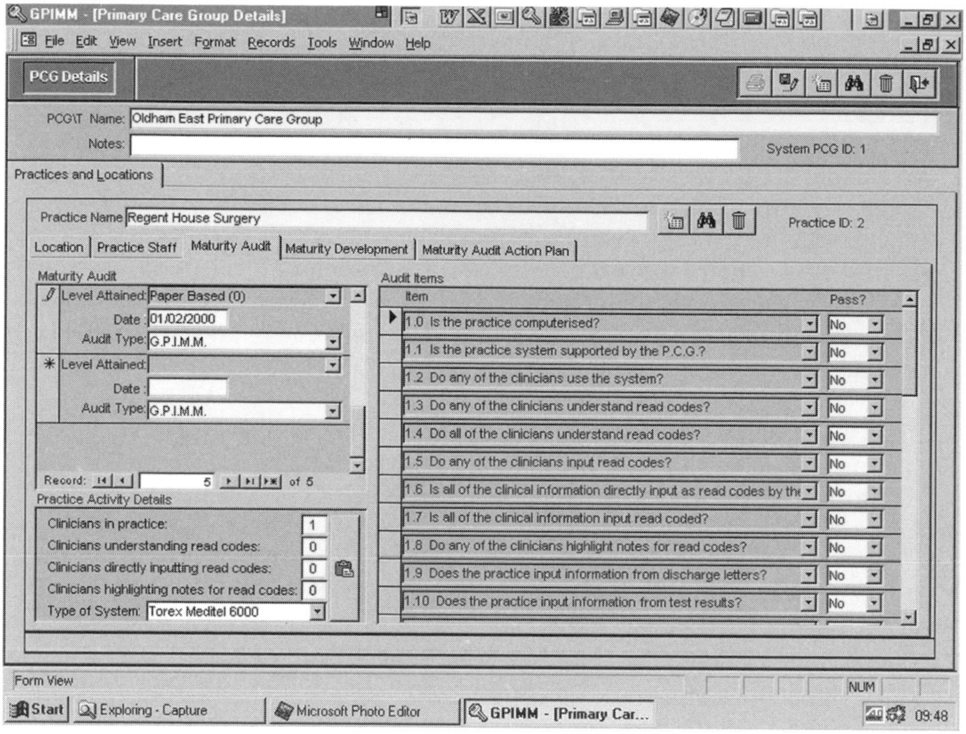

Figure 10.1 Survey of practice computerisation.

capability of each person is that required to meet the needs of the organisation. A similar computerised survey tool can be used to survey training needs (*see* Figure 10.3) and to construct a training programme (*see* Figure 10.4).

What can be achieved

The key to using information is to integrate it as part of the interactive process of care.[12] Roper and Cutler suggest that there are three requirements for systems to work effectively.[13]

1 They should produce information that is valued by healthcare consumers, purchasers and providers.
2 There should be sufficient standardisation in measurement to enable valid comparisons to be made.
3 The measures should be amenable to efficient data collection processes in order to minimise costs.

There are two types of obstacle to achieving these aims – technical and procedural. There needs to be a balance between measuring the (technically) measurable and measuring the (procedurally) meaningful.

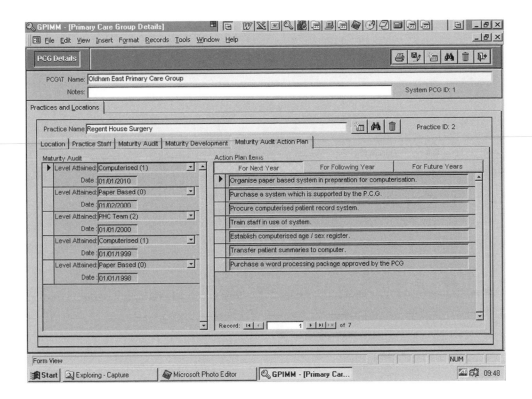

Figure 10.2   Structured action plan.

Table 10.2   Training needs matrix

	GP	Nurse	Manager	Administrator
Competency 1	Required level	Required level	Required level	Required level
Competency 2	Required level	Required level	Required level	Required level
Competency 3	Required level	Required level	Required level	Required level
Competency 4	Required level	Required level	Required level	Required level
Competency 5	Required level	Required level	Required level	Required level

Primary healthcare professionals have traditionally organised their clinical communications in different ways, including free text, coded data (e.g. Read codes) and the use of structured templates that facilitate data entry (e.g. for hypertensive patients). There has been no widespread agreement about what should be recorded, how or why. Consequently, there is considerable variation in the way in which clinical information is structured and stored. These variations are of two main types:

- *structural* – how the information is organised (e.g. free text, coded, coded and supplemented by free text, and so on)

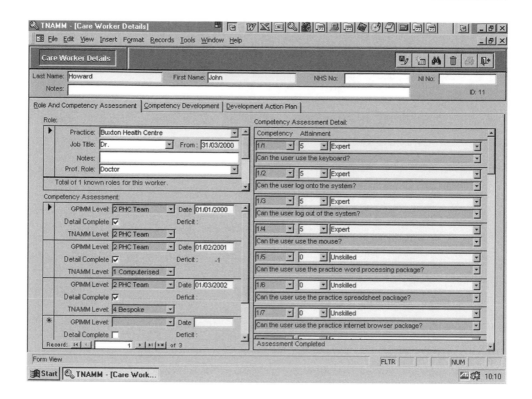

Figure 10.3 Survey of training needs.

- *behavioural* – the consistency with which the information is organised and recorded.

The use of standard coding policies needs a developmental approach to ensure changes in behaviour and ultimately consistency among multiprofessional groups, so that the various and multifaceted requirements can be met over time. Here we shall consider what might be involved in developing the consistent organisation and sharing of information about health and management of a given condition at a given point in time. With an increasing emphasis on monitoring the quality of patient care, and the development of more complex forms of multiprofessional working, the need for consistency in the recording and extraction of data is self-evident. Equally, education and training to support improvement in clinical communications are essential if primary care trusts are to satisfy individual and organisational information needs.

If it is to be fit for its purpose, any framework for managing information should be determined by the requirements of clinical care, ensuring that core clinical information is recorded during individual interventions. The time taken to find information in individual records should decrease, as standardised data recording ensures the immediate availability of core information. It is important to note that seamless methods of data extraction do not remove the clinical responsibility to

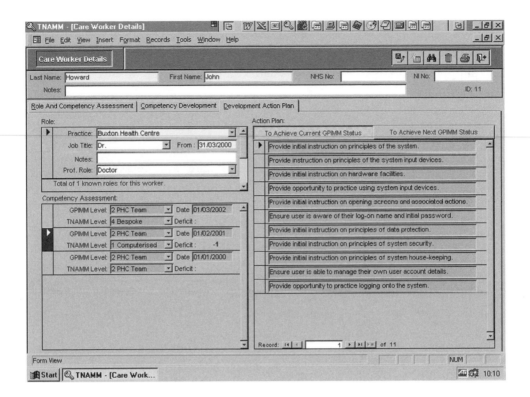

Figure 10.4 Training action plan.

validate the information, and to develop trust and understanding of roles across professional boundaries.

Effective communication is the essential ingredient for developing a culture that is conducive to quality improvement, and it should be two-way, open and designed to generate trust. The care of the patient or client should remain paramount, regardless of organisational structures. Ultimately information should be available from systems to meet core requirements to support the following related processes:

- clinical audit
- performance improvement and review
- accountability
- public health data for monitoring health improvement, needs assessment and service planning
- electronic health records to support the 24-hour provision of care.

The development should be based on team decisions, clearly identifying the necessity for commitment within teams to manage their own performance. The next section will examine the processes involved in establishing a coding policy in a primary care trust to allow the measurement, monitoring, benchmarking and evaluation of service delivery in line with national priorities and standards, while at the same time being responsive to local needs. Communication channels should be established creatively and simply to ensure inclusivity. Dedicated facilitation and support are necessary for clinical staff to gain ownership of the development of the process.

Developing consistency in recording

The development process begins with multidisciplinary dialogue to allow identification of and agreement on the standards to be adopted for monitoring purposes. Discussion should start by considering the care that the team feels should be provided for their patients or clients. The professionals must feel that they have been instrumental, in partnership with patients and carers, in describing the appropriate care and standards of service for their patients and clients, if there is to be confidence in the subsequent extraction of information for monitoring, benchmarking or the evaluation of clinical performance. Ideally, data extraction should use the potential of technology so that system users can access, assemble, aggregate and analyse data held within electronic patient records maintained through the routine provision of care.

The reliability of the information that is derived from the records will depend on the consistency and completeness of those records. It is important that systems provide facilities to enable suitable data entry at the point of care delivery. The true benefits of electronic health records can only be delivered if those records play an active role in the delivery of care. The aim should be to 'work smarter', not to duplicate effort by providing information more than once. If structured data have been recorded, suitable software should enable the extraction of that data to provide information for those who require it. Health professionals should be encouraged to take ownership and harness the potential of emerging technology effectively.

Different practices or teams will have different approaches, skills, interests and mixes of patients. They will need to be facilitated and guided to ensure consistency of core data components, while at the same time being allowed to develop an individual response to implementation to suit their working environment. The elements include the following:

- dialogue between multidisciplinary team members to determine specific selection criteria and content of the information to be extracted from individual patient records
- identification of the prevalence of particular morbidities and changes over time
- monitoring of levels and types of activities
- progress towards health-gain targets for specified patient groups
- compliance with National Service Frameworks
- review of the achievement of expected outcomes.

The process should be dynamic and capable of being reviewed and refined as necessary. Comparison of different types of measures between clinicians, practices and primary care trusts benchmarked against local and national data will highlight areas for investigation or action. MIQUEST is a tool for extracting data from primary care clinical systems.*

Managing information across a primary care trust

Healthcare professionals have traditionally organised their clinical communications in a multitude of different ways. To create a robust primary care trust information standard, the following factors need to be considered:

- appreciation of the way in which professional groups and organisations behave and communicate
- the characteristics of paper- and computer-based health record systems
- standards of system design and architecture.

Ideally, the primary care trust should use an improvement programme consisting of the following steps repeated at intervals:

1 an initial survey to establish a baseline of current activity and consistency of recording standard codes
2 validation of results by each individual practice
3 the production of an improvement plan for each individual practice
4 a repeat survey to determine to what extent the plan has succeeded, and a subsequent repeat of the whole process to ensure that there is continuous improvement.

Practices will need to provide information about their populations, to identify specific target groups of patients, to describe their current delivery of care (including details of which staff perform which tasks) and to identify areas which they feel that they need to address. In particular, they will need to specify the following:

- which staff will do the work
- what extra time this will take
- what additional administration will be needed
- whether the tasks will be undertaken in formal clinics or opportunistically
- how the information will be recorded and how the practice will ensure that the information is accurately and consistently coded
- what systems of recall will be developed
- which guidelines or frameworks will be used.

Figures 10.5, 10.6 and 10.7 set out a three-step approach.

*Support for the use of MIQUEST is provided by the PRIMIS project. PRIMIS is an NHS Information Authority-funded project that provides training and support for local information needs (*see* www. primis.nhs.uk/).

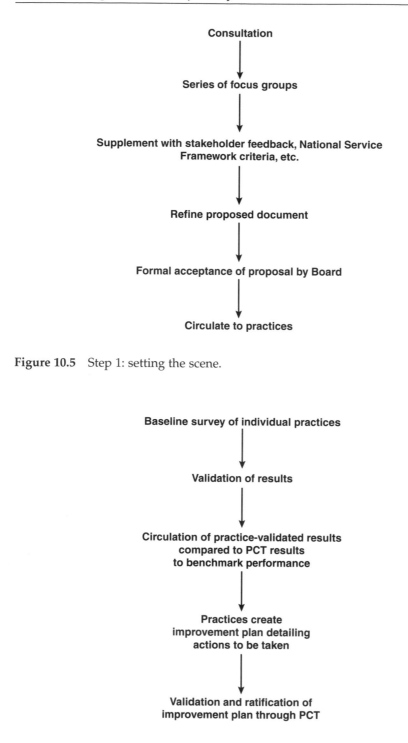

Figure 10.5 Step 1: setting the scene.

Figure 10.6 Step 2: audit/benchmarking/improvement plan.

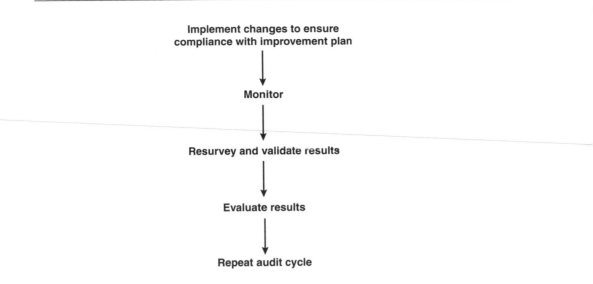

Figure 10.7   Step 3: implementation, monitoring, evaluation and repeat.

Table 10.3 provides an example of a survey of a practice, and Table 10.4 provides an example of a survey of a primary care trust (Fylde Primary Care Trust).
    The aims of the exercise with Fylde Primary Care Trust were as follows:

- to recognise patients with pre-existing coronary heart disease as a percentage of the practice population (G3), and to show a reduction in the levels of those risk factors that have been demonstrated to reduce disability and death, and an increase in treatments that have been demonstrated to do likewise
- to provide accurate and comparable computer-coded information about the treatment of patients with coronary heart disease.[14]

The ways in which practices make improvements vary from one practice to another, but examples include the following:

- implementing a disease management framework that satisfies National Service Framework criteria and local health need requirements
- focusing on specific coded disease topics (e.g. G3)
- standardising risk factor coding (e.g. ex-smoker, heavy smoker, aspirin prophylaxis – to include those patients who purchase their prescriptions over the counter from a pharmacist)
- using electronic laboratory links for comparable coding and sharing of cholesterol results across primary and secondary care.

National policy developments

The National Service Framework for Coronary Heart Disease was published after the work with Fylde Primary Care Trust had been completed. It provided for the

Table 10.3 A practice survey

Practice audit results	Read/BNF code	Age range (years)				Total
		<45	46–60	61–75	>75	
1 All patients in practice		6405	2280	1333	706	10 724
2 All patients with coronary heart disease or atrial fibrillation	G3/G573	5	71	191	141	408
From this subgroup:						
3 Patients with recorded myocardial infarction	G30/G31/G32	3	27	76	54	160
4 Patients with recorded coronary artery surgery	792	2	15	39	8	64
5 Current smokers	137R	1	17	25	11	54
6 Current non-smokers	137L	3	53	163	126	345
7 Aspirin prescribed in last 2 months	BNF2.9/4.7.1			124	87	211
8 Anticoagulant prescribed in last 2 months	BNF 2.8	1	7	31	11	50
9 Adverse reaction to aspirin	TJ53.1					
10 Ever had cholesterol test recorded	44P	4	66	186		256
11 Ever had LDL-cholesterol >3.1 mmol/l recorded	44P6	0	14	44		58
12 Latest LDL-cholesterol recorded <3.1 mmol/l	44P6	2	13	21		36
13 Lipid-lowering drugs prescribed in last 2 months	BNF 2.12	3	44	115	24	186
14 Ever had blood pressure recorded	2469/246A	5	71	191	140	407
15 Ever had systolic blood pressure >140 mmHg or diastolic blood pressure >85 mmHg	2469/246A	3	67	187	140	397
16 Latest systolic blood pressure <140 mmHg and diastolic blood pressure <85 mmHg	2469/246A	5	21	52	28	106
17 Nitrates and/or digoxin prescribed in last 2 months	BNF 2.6.1/2.1	2	26	96	106	230

first time national standards to support integrated care. Successive National Service Frameworks have increasingly defined common information requirements for the key clinical areas.

Table 10.4   Survey of Fylde Primary Care Trust

Fylde Primary Care Trust initial audit	Read/BNF code	Age range (years)				
		<45	46–60	61–75	>75	Total
All patients with coronary heart disease or atrial fibrillation	G3/G573	0.1%	2.7%	12.9%	18.3%	4.9%
From this subgroup:						
Current smokers	137R	39%	19.6%	10.5%	5.5%	9.8%
Current non-smokers	137L	42.3%	59.5%	72.2%	66.5%	68.3%
Aspirin prescribed in last 2 months	BNF2.9/ 4.7.1			60.2%	55.7%	58.2%
Ever had cholesterol test recorded	44P	51.8%	66.4%	63.6%		63.7%
Ever had LDL-cholesterol >3.1 mmol/l recorded	44P6	5.6%	12.5%	13.3%		12.7%
Latest LDL-cholesterol recorded <3.1 mmol/l	44P6	7.5%	12.6%	12.6%		12.9%
Ever had blood pressure recorded	2469/246A	85.7%	92.8%	89.2%	82.1%	86.4%
Ever had systolic blood pressure >140 mmHg or diastolic blood pressure >85 mmHg	2469/246A	41.6%	61.5%	70.8%	67.2%	67.6%
Latest systolic blood pressure <140 mmHg and diastolic blood pressure <85 mmHg	2469/246A	68.2%	43.7%	40.7%	32.8%	38.3%

The recent draft national specification for an integrated care records service provides further detail and a vision for the future.[15] It defines the following principles for information management and clinical governance.

- Clinical governance and audit of processes and outcomes will take place within individual service providers, with comparisons at practice, primary care trust, care community, strategic health authority and national levels. Audit will also take place of multidisciplinary care pathways and processes which span individual service providers within a care community. Services must enable data to be abstracted from the individual patient records supporting direct care and analysed at all of these levels.
- Systems should enable information to be abstracted from individual patient records to enable audit of each service component's own population of patients with, for example, diabetes (i.e. by individual practices, departments within trusts and specialist services).

- Systems should enable data to be abstracted and assembled on a pan-community basis to enable clinical governance and audit at primary care trust level. Systems should be able to maintain and manage data, enable analysis, and have the functionality to present and deliver information to individuals within organisations with a clinical governance role and to feed back information to clinicians about their own services.
- Access to comparative information is needed (e.g. national and other relevant baseline trends and rates) to enable benchmarking of results. Systems should support audit of both processes and outcomes.

Realising such a vision presents an enormous challenge.

Practical points

- Information has a vital role to play in clinical governance.
- The information component must be integrated into the entire process from patient consultation through to monitoring and improvement.
- In order to deliver this information it is necessary to have appropriate technology, processes and human capability.
- Current strategy should deliver technology to support this activity across the NHS over the next five years.
- It remains to be seen whether the organisational systems and human capacity can match the vision for the benefit of patients.

References

1 Gillies AC (2003) *What is a Good Healthcare System?* Radcliffe Medical Press, Oxford.
2 Donaldson L (1999) *Whistleblowing and Clinical Governance.* Speech given at a British Medical Association/*British Medical Journal* conference on 'Whistleblowing: changing the way we work', London, 10 December 1999.
3 Department of Trade and Industry (1998) *Guide to the Public Interest Disclosure Act.* The Stationery Office, London.
4 Department of Health (1989) *Medical Audit. NHS Review Working Paper 6.* Department of Health, London.
5 Department of Health (1990) *Medical Audit: guidance for hospital clinicians on the use of computers.* Department of Health, London.
6 Scally G and Donaldson LJ (1998) Clinical governance and the drive for quality improvement in the new NHS in England. *BMJ.* **317**: 61–5.
7 Kelson M and Redpath L (1996) Promoting user involvement in clinical audit: surveys of audit committees in primary and secondary care. *J Clin Effect.* **1**: 14–18.
8 Department of Health (1992) *An IM&T Strategy for the National Health Service.* HMSO, London.
9 Department of Health Information Policy Unit (2003) *Delivering Twenty-First Century IT Support for the NHS: national strategic programme.* The Stationery Office, London.

10 Humphrey WS (1989) *Managing the Software Process*. Addison-Wesley, Reading, MA.
11 Dreyfus SE and Dreyfus HL (1980) *A Five-Stage Model of the Mental Activities Involved in Directed Skill Acquisition*. Unpublished report supported by the US Air Force Office of Scientific Research (Contract F49620-79-C-0063). University of California, Berkeley, CA.
12 Knight B (2000) Using information to support different ways of working. In: W Abbott, J Bryant and S Bullas (eds) *Current Perspectives in Health Informatics*. Health Informatics Committee, British Computer Society, London.
13 Roper W and Cutler C (1998) Health plan accountability and reporting. Issues and challenges. *Health Affairs*. **17**: 152–5.
14 Hardwick SA and Mechan J (2000) How Fylde PCG put practices at the heart of its CHD plan. In: *Vision Doctor* (Supplement). Reed Healthcare Publishing, London.
15 Department of Health Information Policy Unit (2003) *Delivering Twenty-First Century IT Support for the NHS: draft national specification for integrated care records service* (version 1.2f). The Stationery Office, London.

CHAPTER 11

Reducing risk and promoting safety in primary care

Tim Wilson* and Stephen Rogers

First do no harm.

Attributed to Hippocrates

> This chapter explains the definitions surrounding risk and introduces the concept of patient safety. The specific areas of activity in primary care where patient safety is at risk are described, and techniques that have been used successfully in other industries to analyse and minimise risk are explored.

Safety is everybody's business, and clinicians and managers alike need to consider whether the actions they take are the best ones for the patient. Safety has champions (clinical governance leads, clinical directors, and executive and non-executive directors) whose mission is to promote safer care. This chapter then is for everyone, but we would especially commend it to the 'champions'.

Introduction

Everyone involved with clinical governance in primary care should take heed of the Hippocratic quote at the beginning of the chapter. For there is evidence that we are harming our patients, and this should not be the case. The duty of clinical governance leads in primary care organisations and in practices, of primary care organisation chief executives and their boards, of professional executive committees and of every individual working in primary care is clear – to reduce harm. There are both legal and professional reasons for this, but above all else this needs to come from the heart. This needs passion. We would argue that primary care organisations should charge a senior non-executive board member with the responsibility for asking the difficult safety questions at every opportunity.

---

*Tim Wilson is a policy analyst at the Department of Health, but the views expressed in this chapter are his own.

Just as medical progress increases our ability to help patients, so it seems to increase the potential for harm. Clinicians are increasingly recognising the importance of ensuring patient safety (clinical risk management), although it is not a new problem. Their attention seems to have been captured by high-profile cases of error, theme issues of medical journals, and perhaps also by Government publications.

Our understanding of safety in primary care is growing,[1] but there is still a long way to go. This poses a real challenge for the National Patient Safety Agency (*see* below and www.npsa.nhs.uk).[2] The scale of serious harm in primary care is probably of the order of 0.2% per episode of care. However, the volume of consultations in primary care means that the overall level of patient harm might be high, albeit uncommon in any one practice. This poses a particular difficulty for primary care – it is difficult to plan for rare events.

However, we can anticipate matters becoming worse as primary care becomes increasingly complex. Conditions that were previously the province of the hospital specialist are now firmly established in primary care. Early hospital discharge is the norm. Prescribing and monitoring of potentially dangerous drugs is commonplace, and polypharmacy is now officially sanctioned for patients (often the elderly) with ischaemic heart disease and diabetes. Finally, there is the pressure of short consultations. In a recent editorial in the *British Medical Journal* it was pointed out that more research is needed.[3] This is true, but waiting for the results of studies to become available will mean that patients will be harmed in the interim by action or inaction that is *known* to be less safe.

We also need to ask ourselves whether the newer term 'patient safety' is merely fashionable. Why is the medical world taking safety seriously when risk management has been around for years? Risk management does have connotations of risk avoidance that patient safety does not. Safety 'feels' as if it is a whole-system issue (patient, clinician, administration, management and leadership), whereas risk management has sometimes been perceived (by clinicians at least) as a problem for management. The word 'safety' seems to have captured patient and clinician attention in a manner that risk management did not.

That we are entering a period of activity to improve safety, where risk management seemed to have little impact, is a development to be welcomed. However, the lessons learned from risk management, and in particular the expertise of those involved, should not be lost. Fortunately, the leading proponents in the field of risk management are in the forefront of the safety movement. Furthermore, risk management does have implications for the health and safety of employees in organisations that *patient* safety does not.[4]

The National Patient Safety Agency (NPSA) is working on a number of fronts to reduce harm. Key parts of their remit include developing a reporting system and spreading effective methods for the investigation of incidents (a more detailed outline of the proposed work of the NPSA is shown in Boxes 11.1 and 11.2).

Box 11.1   Goals for the National Patient Safety Agency

1 Local reporting of adverse events and action to reduce risk within the organisation concerned are essential.
2 On a selective basis, reports to national level will enable service-wide action where patterns, clusters or trends reveal the scope to reduce risk or prevent recurrence for future patients in other parts of the country.
3 The necessary steps that need to be taken to set up the linked components of the new system include the following:
   • establishing agreed definitions of adverse events and near misses
   • building expertise in root cause analysis within the NHS
   • ensuring that there is pooling of information from all other major existing adverse-event-reporting systems
   • promoting a culture of reporting and patient safety within NHS organisations
   • where risks are identified, producing solutions to prevent harm, specifying national goals and establishing mechanisms to track progress
   • reducing the incidence of multiple inspections and accreditation visits by rationalising the current system
   • giving patients and carers a role in the adverse-event-reporting system
   • addressing staff concerns about standards of care by implementing the new adverse-event-reporting system, and continuing to protect staff by whistleblowing legislation.
4 Specific risks targeted for action:
   • reduce by 25% by 2005 the number of instances of harm in the field of obstetrics and gynaecology which result in litigation
   • reduce by 40% by 2005 the number of serious errors in the use of prescribed drugs.

Box 11.2   Further goals for the National Patient Safety Agency

Other areas that have been identified where action by the NPSA could provide some early gains in risk reduction include the following:

• review of the care environment to identify environmental changes and changes in care practices that could reduce risk and improve patient safety
• review of clinical practice with Royal Colleges, professional organisations and specialist associations to identify high-risk procedures
• building safety into purchasing policy within the NHS
• seeking input from the world of design to identify new opportunities for improved safety
• examining across the board the potential for computers to reduce the occurrence and impact of error

- identifying the scope for formal pre-procedure safety briefings in very high-risk situations
- enhancing the role of simulation laboratories in exposing staff to risk situations where there are no actual patients involved
- creating a clear role for patients in helping to promote and achieve safety goals.

Terminology and semantics

Semantics is important because words convey meaning. If we want to communicate the importance of safety in clinical governance, we need to use the right language.[5]

The terms 'error', 'mistake' and 'preventable' are largely unhelpful if your goal is to improve patient care. Error and mistake both imply that someone has done something wrong, yet we know that humans will make mistakes roughly 4% of the time when performing routine or repetitive tasks. To suggest that those who work in healthcare should 'try harder' is misguided and has not stood the test of time. However, it is useful to acknowledge mistakes and errors when they occur. They are learning opportunities, and above all else they are clarion calls for change. In making an error someone is not necessarily wrong – they are only at fault if they do not act afterwards (*see* section below on learning from adverse events).

We are said to be entering a 'no-blame culture', but some are now talking about 'fair blame'. Does this mean that we can breathe a sigh of relief? For most, actions will speak louder than words, and we will be convinced when there is system-wide (including Government, media and societal) support for teams acting to learn from an incident. Airline industries protect employees from disciplinary action if they report an error (but not if they are malicious). With the right of protection when trying to learn from harm comes a heavy responsibility – we have to act when we know that there is a problem. Failure to do so should result in blame.

Preventable and non-preventable adverse events are ambiguous terms. If a patient has a haemorrhage while on warfarin (e.g. is admitted with an epistaxis), is this one of the expected and so non-preventable outcomes of therapy? Possibly, but it is only non-preventable if every possible means has been taken to prevent it (e.g. using the best system for monitoring, education and patient involvement). The boundary between preventable and non-preventable outcomes is largely determined by what we deem to be acceptable and affordable. Although there are examples at the extremes (e.g. the first allergic reaction is clearly not preventable, but subsequent reactions are), most events are less clearly preventable or non-preventable.

Significant, critical or adverse events obviously need to be defined, mainly for the purposes of the mandatory national reporting system. Everyone involved will need to know what to report and what not to report. Definitions are less important for the purpose of analysis of events on a local basis, except for the purposes of maximising learning across all activities of the organisation. Something is an important event if you (or more appropriately your patient) think it is (*see* discussion of learning events in Chapter 4).

Some experts talk about direct, contributory and latent causes of adverse events. Direct causes describe those actions or events that had an immediate link to the event (e.g. dispensing the wrong medication). Direct events are often due to human frailties, so should be anticipated at a rate of around 4% (*see* below for a discussion of the error rate of dispensing medication), and can be avoided by good design – not castigation. Contributory causes are other factors that led up to the problem (e.g. the pharmacist was distracted by a phone call), and again they can be avoided by paying attention to the environment and the conditions in which the event occurred. Latent causes are those that have only a distant but nevertheless potent link with the adverse event. Consider the following fictitious example. A chain of commercial high-street chemists extend their pharmacists' roles so that in addition to dispensing prescriptions they are also expected to deal with telephone enquiries. This increases the possibility of a dispensing error. Indeed, the error made on 3 July by a pharmacist in Wokingham, who dispensed the wrong strength of digoxin, was directly linked to the decision in the boardroom eight months previously.

Any adverse event is likely to be the final step in a chain of actions. At each step of that chain there is the potential to detect the problem and then prevent the adverse event from occurring. Adverse events therefore only occur when there is a failure to spot the problem at every stage of the process. In primary care, the most obvious case is where the pharmacist misses the prescribing error by the GP, which has already been missed by the GP's computer and the pharmacist's computer. This is often referred to as the Swiss cheese model (alluding to the many holes in Swiss cheese, and how those holes have to be aligned before something can pass through the layers of cheese). However, it is worth remembering that models are only models, and some would argue that 'all models are useful, but all models are wrong'.[6]

'Patient safety' and 'patient harm' are the most useful terms as they simply describe what they are – times when patient care is safe or when harm has been done. When we grapple with safety and harm then we are attempting to make the system better.

The specific problem of safety in primary care

There are features of primary care (*see* Box 11.3) which enhance patient safety, but there are also areas of activity where safety is particularly at risk. The latter category includes the following:

- prescribing
- communication
- organisation
- diagnosis.

Box 11.3   Strengths of general practice

With some exceptions, UK general practice:

- is strongly team based
- has good continuity of care
- has consistent and longitudinal records
- uses computerised prescribing
- includes a pharmacist in the dispensing of medicines
- pays close attention to the concerns of patients (ideas, concerns and expectations)
- often uses significant audit (perhaps 20% of practices on a regular basis)
- is beginning to develop a stronger co-operative model across practices (out-of-hours co-operatives and primary care trust-wide quality initiatives).

Prescribing

Perhaps because of its nature, prescribing has been most intensively researched with regard to safety. Prescribing problems in general practice occur at a rate of between 3% and 5% of all prescriptions, of which about one-third can be classified as having major safety concerns (i.e. about 1% in total).

A quarter of the claims against GP members of the Medical Defence Union in 1996 related to medication safety issues. Common themes to emerge included prescription of contraindicated medication, dispensing errors, ignoring known allergies or simply prescribing the wrong drug. In an Australian study, around 9% of hospital admissions were considered to be due to potentially avoidable medication problems. Although safety considerations are important with all prescribed treatments, there are particular safety issues with certain drug classes, namely non-steroidal anti-inflammatory drugs (NSAIDs), lithium, warfarin, corticosteroids and antidepressants. Around 1% of patients over 75 years of age who are taking an NSAID without gastric protection will have a major haemorrhage. Dispensing of drugs by pharmacists is another source of error. In one US-based study, it was calculated that over the course of a year 4% of drugs were incorrectly dispensed.

For a more detailed review of prescribing issues in primary care, the reader is directed to the *British Journal of General Practice* Quality Supplement.[7]

Communication

Communication breakdown is a common cause of patient harm. However, it is more often a symptom of organisational problems than a cause. In some cases, communication breakdown has resulted from the informality of the communication process. A forgotten comment in the surgery corridor or a Post-it note that fell behind a desk are everyday occurrences with which all clinicians will readily identify (P Lambden, personal communication, 2001). Transcription of information (e.g. when dictating referral letters) and the associated risk of inaccuracy represents another important source of communication error.

Perhaps most alarming is the transition between hospital and the community, with discrepancies being found for around 40% of patients between the drugs prescribed at the point of discharge and the drugs they receive at home. Deaths have occurred because patients took the hospital-supplied medicines *and* the supply they had previously obtained from their GP. This situation is especially likely to occur if different names are used (e.g. generic name on one and proprietary name on another). This is an issue that requires system-wide improvement between sectors.

Organisation

Most pronouncements on safety have emphasised the importance of developing the 'right' organisational culture. However, there is little research evidence with regard to the desirable cultural characteristics for safety in primary care. It is not even known, for example, whether culture is something that can be determined or managed in healthcare. However, there has been research in industry, specifically the aviation industry, and empirical evidence from evaluation of the role of teamwork, communication and leadership suggests that untoward incidents can be reduced. We are in no doubt that some cultural characteristics are 'toxic' to care. Failure of senior leaders to support teams, or to work on improving safety, and poor relationships between staff have all been shown to lead to poor patient outcomes.[8]

Diagnosis

In one anonymous study, diagnostic problems accounted for 28% of reported errors, of which 50% were considered to be potentially very harmful. Failure to diagnose in time is the major cause of complaints in defence society databases (65%). The overall frequency of diagnostic errors in primary care is unknown.

Conditions that appear to be particularly problematic (or where it is easier to find a misdiagnosis with hindsight) include asthma, cancer, dermatological conditions, substance abuse and depression. One in every 29 GP consultations is reported to include a case of missed depression. Overall, missed fractures are the commonest cause of litigation.

Any review of the wide range of referral patterns in primary care highlights the difficulties clinicians experience in making diagnoses. Some health policy makers and managers might regard high referral rates as inefficient, yet 'failure to refer appropriately' is a major contributory factor in many successful claims against general practitioners.

Reliable organisations and culture

It has been said that just as medicine knows more about disease than about health, so science knows more about what causes adverse events than about how they can be avoided. This is not entirely the case. Studies of organisations that need to be extremely reliable, but which like healthcare are complex, with multiple human inputs, have shown a number of specific organisational characteristics.[9] We have mentioned the need for strong leadership in the field of safety. Two additional characteristics that are important for healthcare are anticipating problems and containing problems.

Leadership

The importance of leadership cannot be over-emphasised, and it is a particular responsibility of primary care organisation chief executives, directors, clinical governance leads and primary care team leaders (*see*, for example, the role of the executive partner in Chapter 4) to ensure patient safety.

Anticipating problems

Healthcare teams should never assume that everything is fine, because it rarely is. Reliable organisations are preoccupied with safety – they constantly check, observe and review. Furthermore, they are reluctant to simplify when problems do occur. They look for the cause (*see* below) and deal with it. They understand that when things go wrong this is usually due to a complex set of interactions. Lastly, they are sensitive to performance. They have systems for monitoring performance, and respond as soon as something appears to be going wrong. Far from having a mandatory *reporting* system (as is proposed in the NHS for England), they have a mandatory *responding* system.

Containing problems

Reliable organisations are committed to resilience. Not only do they have mechanisms for detecting problems at an early stage, but they also have systems in place for mitigating any further deterioration. There are many components to this, but an important principle in healthcare is deferring to the real expert. Often parents or carers will tell healthcare workers when something is going wrong. The healthcare system needs to ensure that it is able to respond to these 'expert' concerns.

Improvement and design

In medicine, the task that faces managers and clinicians, especially clinical governance leads, is to improve or redesign the systems which permit errors to occur. By 'system' we mean the equipment, dressings or drugs involved, the processes and procedures adopted, and the activities of the healthcare professionals involved in providing the care.

Diagnosing system problems

In high-risk industries outside healthcare, such as the aerospace industry, assurance of safe functioning is a prerequisite before any system is commissioned. In medicine, some systems exist as organisational habits, or have evolved with insufficient emphasis on patient safety. Such systems are unlikely to deliver satisfactory outcomes for patients. Some of them have built-in design faults which put patients at risk.

Assessment of the degree of risk associated with an existing or new system or technology is known as *failure analysis*. A safe system requires perfect synergy between technology, humans, procedures, management and administrative functions. The process of failure analysis identifies problem areas in a system and provides the opportunity to introduce measures for error reduction and error detection.

Failure analysis typically draws on tools and techniques that belong to the armamentarium of continuous quality improvement.[10,11] These approaches are new to many in healthcare, but are gaining ground fast. Process flow diagrams can be drawn to help us to understand how patients, materials or information move between compartments in the healthcare process. Cause-and-effect charts can help health workers to understand the causes of problems that might occur during the delivery of care. Matrix graphs can be used to prioritise areas that require immediate attention, by flagging errors that have a high risk of occurrence and/or potentially serious implications for patients.

The matrix graph is central to risk assessments conducted in practices.[12] The typical scenario is for an outside 'expert' to visit the practice and to convene an interactive meeting with practice staff to identify which aspects of practice are most likely to generate problems, and to assess how serious those problems could conceivably be. The results of such assessments then provide the starting point for practice staff to introduce changes or controls which might be expected to reduce the frequency of problems or allow their detection before they lead to adverse outcomes. Box 11.4 shows an example of a matrix graph for use in primary care. In each cell the primary care team can assess the likely risks and prioritise them according to their likely frequency, level of harm and potential for prevention (e.g. patients/prescribing – patients taking too much or too little prescribed medication, communication/hospitals – hospital discharge letters failing to provide sufficient or accurate information).

Box 11.4 Risk matrix graph

Risks/Sources	Patients	Practice health professionals	Practice ancillary staff	Hospitals
Prescribing				
Communication				
Organisation				
Diagnosis				

Design principles for safer systems

There are some principles of design that can be used to make systems safer[13] (*see* Box 11.5). Applying these techniques is often the clue to designing safer systems, and so offers the means to address problems identified by systems analysis.

Box 11.5   Design principles for safer systems

Simplification is about reducing complexity. Many clinical activities are complex, but some are made so unnecessarily. Increasing standardisation and reducing unnecessary alternatives, such as agreeing to adopt a practice drug formulary, is an example of simplification.

Automation of processes can reduce errors provided that it is used wisely and to assist rather than to supplant the human operator. Use of computers in repeat prescribing is associated with a substantial reduction in prescribing errors.

Reminders such as checklists, protocols and templates can optimise information processing and help preserve available short-term memory for communication and problem solving during a consultation.

Affordances are prompts (usually visual) that guide the user. Providing different-coloured containers for bottle banks for disposal of green, brown and plain glass bottles is an example.

Constraints are barriers that have to be overcome in order to complete an action. Not being able to remove money from a cash machine until you have removed your cash card is a very effective means of preventing cards from being forgotten.

Differentiation involves sorting different items into different categories so that confusion should never occur. In healthcare an example of this might be keeping anaesthetics containing adrenaline well away from other anaesthetics.

Repetition is used by nursing staff who are administering a parenteral drug. The action of checking the drug, dose and expiry date is repeated.

Minimising handoff involves trying to avoid transcription errors. These can be prevented by using automatic transfer of data so that information does not have to be transcribed repeatedly.

Closing the quality circle

Not every change leads to an improvement. Desirable outcomes do not always follow changes that have been made with the best intentions. Continuous quality improvement offers a systematic, planned approach to quality improvement and is applicable to problems of patient safety, as well as to clinical effectiveness and operational efficiency. Measurement of the impact of a change is one of the key underpinning features of continuous quality improvement thinking. Infrequent, serious adverse events are not amenable to monitoring in quality improvement cycles, but errors or other deviations from the ideal may be specified and monitored. The successful application of continuous quality improvement approaches to organisational problems such as appointment systems, telephone messages and repeat prescribing has been demonstrated in primary care.[14] Patients being unable to consult with the doctor when they are ill, telephone messages becoming mislaid or patients' prescriptions not being ready on time are quality problems, which can have implications for patient safety.

For more information on some of these techniques the reader is directed to the leadership guides which are available free from the Modernisation Agency (www. modern.nhs.uk), and to the resources available from the National Patient Safety Agency (www.npsa.org.uk).

Learning from error

Learning from errrors is crucial. Everyone in primary care should be participating in activities that are directed towards understanding what happened when something went wrong, and preventing the same thing from occurring in the future. This might take the form of reflecting on problems when they occur, or participating in multidisciplinary meetings to review and analyse a series of problems which have occurred in particular settings. Alternatively, for a more serious event or series of events, primary care staff may be invited to participate in an inquiry led by the primary care organisation.

Every healthcare worker (and risk manager!) should know something about the following approaches which may be used to learn from errors in the delivery of healthcare.

Local reporting of incidents with implications for patient safety is to become obligatory for healthcare professionals working in the NHS. Any reporting system will allow for a description of the clinical scenario, the nature and severity of the outcome, and the story of what happened, and will probably ask for contributory causes and the corrective action required. Completing a report form will encourage reflection on the part of the individual reporting – and might require consideration and action by a wider group – as well as providing essential information for primary care organisations and national efforts to monitor aspects of patient safety. The report is likely to be based on the memory of an individual who may not have a full understanding of the circumstances surrounding the incident, but it has the advantage that it can be relatively quickly produced.

Critical incident analysis might be considered to be the progenitor of all other approaches. Flanagan pioneered the approach in his early studies of combat veterans by asking them to report on their own and others' behaviour in critical incidents or near misses involving aircraft.[15] In healthcare the same approach is used as an educational tool for encouraging reflection, clarifying and understanding decisions made, and identifying areas of practice that require attention. Incidents may be either collected prospectively or recalled from memory. The story of the incident, good and less good aspects of care and lessons learned can be written down in private, for confidential discussion with a supervisor or mentor. Thus the focus is on personal development and individual learning.

Significant event auditing is already established in many general practice settings. This is a team-based approach to quality assurance, and it may be directed towards clinical and administrative problems with implications for patient safety, clinical effectiveness and patient satisfaction (*see* Chapter 12). Positive aspects of care as well as aspects that need improvement are discussed, and disclosure and frank exchange are encouraged. The process needs to be well managed if it is to be productive, but insights into causes of problems may emerge and can support the generation of action plans. The approach is efficient. A number of events can be considered in sequence, without the need to track down various members of staff, and the individuals who consider the causes are likely to be the people responsible for the implementation of changes.

Organisational cause analysis is an explicit systems-based approach to the investigation of errors and adverse events. Although organisational cause analysis has mainly been used in hospital settings and for more serious adverse events, the approach is certainly applicable to primary care. The inclusion of a framework that prompts consideration of patient factors, staff factors, communication issues, work environment factors and organisational and policy issues helps to identify influences operating at various levels which together have the effect of compromising patient safety. It is argued that the approach leads very naturally to the generation of action plans. Primary care organisations might well use this approach when investigating more serious incidents, but the framework can also be used in small group discussions to ensure that considerations of cause are thorough and systematic.

Root cause analysis is linked to the continuous quality improvement approaches discussed earlier. In this approach an incident or a cluster of incidents precipitates an investigation. The 'What happened?' and 'How did it happen?' questions are addressed, much as in other methods, through group or individual interviews and record review. In addition, diagnostic approaches such as process flow and cause-and-effect diagrams are used to study the systems that are assumed to be at fault. Root cause analysis assumes that chains of events generate adverse events, and an approach that is often used during interviewing is the '5 Ys'. If something happened, then why did it happen? And why did that happen? And why did that happen? And what precipitated that? And so on. Although process flow and cause-and-effect charting will require some practice, and might need to be facilitated, the '5 Ys' can be incorporated into small group discussions as a technique for ensuring that root causes of problems are considered. The full-blown root cause analysis is more likely to be conducted by primary care organisations interested in addressing a particular area of healthcare that has generated a serious event or a series of events judged to be problematic.

Healthcare staff remain concerned about discussing errors and mistakes. Fear of exposure, blame or humiliation is common among people who have arguably been trained to be invincible. They may also have experienced organisational settings in which mistakes were followed by disciplinary action. In multidisciplinary meetings, hierarchical barriers, poor group dynamics or concerns about confidentiality can arise. Even in one-to-one interviews a range of emotional responses can be encountered, ranging from extreme distress to frank denial. The Chief

Medical Officer's report *An Organisation With a Memory* set the scene for the future by describing how the culture of organisations could change to ensure that learning takes place when a mistake is made. Careful communication, confidentiality, an appropriate focus on systems and dissociation of investigations from litigation will all be essential for thorough and meaningful analysis of clinical incidents.

Closing the quality circle (again)

Healthcare workers need to feel that their disclosures and professional time lead to valuable learning that will be translated into improved services for patients. It is important that incident reports do not simply gather dust, but are used to trigger investigations or monitor progress. Investigations must be associated with action plans, and those action plans must be implemented. The value of any changes that are made will depend on the thoroughness of the investigation and the validity of the conclusions that are drawn. The final result will also depend on the capacity of key players to implement change. Not every change leads to an improvement. Safer care does not always follow change, so the impact of change should be measured.

Further reading

- Reason J (2000) Human error: models and management. *BMJ*. **320**: 768–70.
- Institute of Medicine (2000) *To Err is Human: building a safer health system*. Institute of Medicine, USA.
- Vincent C (ed.) (2001) *Clinical Risk Management: enhancing patient safety*. BMJ Books, London.

Useful websites

- www.modern.nhs.uk (website for the Modernisation Agency, with useful redesign and improvement guides)
- www.npsa.org.uk (website for the National Patient Safety Agency, with useful matrices for deciding safety priorities and other tools)
- www.ahrq.org (website for the Agency for Healthcare Research into Quality; it has many useful links to safety, called 'error' on this site)
- www.nelh.nhs.uk (website for the NHS, soon to include a safety and quality section)

Practical points

- There is a new and growing interest in the concept of patient safety, including the establishment of a new national organisation (in England) – the National Patient Safety Agency.
- Human beings make mistakes around 4% of the time when they are undertaking repetitive tasks.
- The scale of serious harm in primary care is around 0.2% per episode of care.
- There are four main areas where patient safety is at risk, namely prescribing, communication, organisation and diagnosis.
- 'Reliable' organisations are preoccupied with safety. They are well led, and both anticipate and contain risks to safety.
- High-risk industries outside healthcare have developed a range of techniques for investigating, preventing and mitigating adverse events.

References

1 Wilson T and Sheikh A (2002) Enhancing public safety in primary care. *BMJ*. **324**: 584–7.
2 Department of Health (2001) *Building a Safer NHS*. The Stationery Office, London.
3 Wilson T, Pringle M and Sheikh A (2001) Promoting safety in primary care. *BMJ*. **323**: 583–4.
4 Wilson T, Smith F and Lakhani M (2002) Patient safety in primary health care – an overview of current developments in risk management and implications for clinical governance. *J Clin Govern*. **10**(1): 25–30.
5 Wilson T and Haraden C (2001) Words, words and more words. *Clin Govern Bull*. **2**(5): 13.
6 Lewin K (1975) *Field Theory in Social Science: selected theoretical papers*. Greenwood Press, Westport, CT.
7 Avery A, Sheikh A, Hurwitz B *et al*. (2002) Safer medicines management in primary care. *Br J Gen Pract*. **52**: s17–22.
8 Rubin I (2000) *Patient Safety and Managerial Malpractice: what's the connection?* Temenos, Hawaii.
9 Weick K and Sutcliffe K (2001) *Managing the Unexpected*. Jossey-Bass, San Francisco, CA.
10 Berwick DM, Godfrey AB and Roessner J (1990) *Curing Health Care*. Jossey Bass, San Francisco, CA.
11 Joint Commission on Accreditation of Healthcare Organizations (2002) *Failure Modes and Effects Analysis in Healthcare: pro-active risk reduction*. JCAHO, Oakbrook Terrace, IL.
12 Standards Association of Australia (1999) *Risk Management AS/NZS 4360:1999*. Standards Association of Australia, Strathfield, NSW.
13 Langley GJ, Nolan KM, Norman CL, Provost LP and Nolan TW (1996) *The Improvement Guide: a practical approach to enhancing organizational performance*. Jossey-Bass, San Francisco, CA.
14 Lawrence M and Packwood T (1996) Adapting total quality management for general practice: evaluation of a programme. *Qual Health Care*. **5**: 151–8.
15 Flanagan J (1954) The critical incident technique. *Psychol Bull*. **51**: 327–58.

CHAPTER 12

Significant event auditing

Mike Pringle

This chapter begins with two clinical cases – straightforward primary care cases – that illustrate the power of significant event auditing. Terms are then defined and the literature is reviewed. Finally, the author describes his personal experience over more than a decade of regular significant event auditing by his primary care team.

Introduction

We all enjoy a good discussion about a patient. We find people and their health-care interesting, and chatting about cases exploits that interest. Sometimes a colleague will say something during such a case discussion that makes us raise our eyebrows. We want to know more, but we feel that we cannot probe without sounding challenging.

Yet locked within these clinical case histories is the richest material – for expanding our knowledge and understanding, for our education and professional development, and for improving care for our patients. The unlocking of that rich seam is called *significant event auditing*.

This technique simply offers a structure for case discussions, giving permission for colleagues to delve and enquire, and for the team to strive together to learn from each other's experience.

Two illustrative cases

The following two cases, in which details have been altered to protect confidentiality, are taken from routine primary care. The first one illustrates the problems of a GP under stress.

Case 1: a urinary infection

Mr Paul Mathews, aged 47, presented urgently at the front desk with frequency and pain on urinating. The receptionist 'fitted him in' with a doctor who was already running half an hour late. The doctor asked for a specimen and saw another patient while Mr Mathews passed urine. The doctor then examined the urine, finding clear evidence of a urinary infection. She prescribed amoxycillin and asked the patient to submit another urine specimen in two weeks' time.

Three days later a colleague was asked to visit Mr Mathews, who had a sustained florid allergic reaction to amoxycillin. Mr Mathews knew that he was allergic to penicillin, but had not been asked specifically about that fact. He had not realised that amoxycillin was a penicillin. The allergy risk was not noted in Mr Mathews' computer record, nor was it written on the cover of the paper record (a previous episode was recorded on a continuation card deep within the paper record). This second partner arranged an X-ray of Mr Mathews' urinary tract. The test demonstrated a mass in the right kidney, which turned out to be a cancer.

Most GPs would recognise two lapses of good medical practice in the above case. First, the possibility of penicillin allergy should be considered whenever a penicillin is to be prescribed. The doctor, who was under pressure, did not ask, but relied on the allergy alert in the computer's prescribing module. In fact the computer record was incomplete because the computer entries had been taken from the front of the manual records, and Mr Mathews' allergy was not recorded on the record envelope.

When the primary care team discussed this case at its significant event meeting, the issue of false reassurance from the computer's failure to alert the doctor (the dog that didn't bark in the night) was raised. The problem of relying on decision support when it fails to support was highlighted. It was agreed the team would ensure that all patients who were prescribed penicillin would be asked about allergies, regardless of whether a computer warning was present.

The second problem was the failure of the doctor to investigate a middle-aged man with a urinary tract infection. The doctor explained that she had intended to start investigations at a subsequent consultation, but no firm arrangement had been made for such an appointment. She agreed to review the literature, and to draft practice guidance on how to handle urinary infections in both men and women of all ages. That protocol was agreed at a later meeting and has been audited regularly since.

The practice discussion moved on to consider doctors' stress and, in particular, the fitting in of extra patients in a busy surgery. This topic recurred regularly over the next six months and culminated in a redesign of the appointments system. The doctor 'on call' for emergencies on any given day would be given protected free appointments in each surgery to enable him or her to cope with patients who could not wait until the end of surgery to be seen.

Thus this one case led to a clinical policy decision, a literature review and new protocol, standard setting for clinical audit and a change in the appointments system!

The second case concerns a complaint where the practice could not defend the care that an elderly patient (who was at considerable risk) had received.

Case 2: a complaint

The practice received a letter of complaint from Mrs Allsop's daughter, Beryl. Beryl had telephoned for a visit for her mother and was told that a doctor would visit. Since no one visited that day, she phoned again the next day and the GP registrar called. He listened carefully to Mrs Allsop's symptoms, examined her thoroughly, and explained that he felt there was 'nothing much the matter'. He arranged for a nurse to visit to take a blood test, which she did that afternoon.

Almost one week later, Beryl became very concerned about her mother and called the surgery on a Saturday afternoon. The duty doctor from the co-operative called and was concerned about Mrs Allsop's breathlessness and pallor. He arranged an emergency admission, and severe anaemia was diagnosed. After transfusion and stopping her arthritis tablets, Mrs Allsop returned home.

The primary care team discussed this case in some detail. First, the reception staff explained the circumstances surrounding the failure to visit. A senior receptionist had taken the message but, having then been immediately distracted, had failed to write it down. After several subsequent meetings with the staff, it was agreed that one receptionist would take all telephone messages – other than requests for appointments – for the first three hours after morning-surgery opening. No visit request has been missed since.

The doctors congratulated the GP registrar on the care that he provided during the home visit. His questioning and examination had been exemplary, and he had arranged an appropriate investigation. Care had fallen down in responding to the faxed result, which had shown a very low haemoglobin value. This result had been placed, with the notes, on the GP registrar's desk. However, he had been absent for a day, and on his return he assumed that action had been taken and that the result was merely there for information.

Clearly something needed to be done to ensure that this situation never recurred. A new policy was agreed whereby all faxed results would go to the duty doctor, who would liaise with the patient's doctor to ensure that appropriate action was taken. The duty doctor would also check all incoming pathology results for any highly abnormal results. It would be this doctor's responsibility to ensure that appropriate action was taken.

The practice manager wrote to Beryl, setting out the content of the practice team's discussion and explaining the actions that had resulted. Beryl visited the practice and discussed her mother's care with the practice manager and one of the doctors. She accepted the full apology of the practice and, in view of the action that the practice had taken, did not pursue a formal complaint.

What do these cases tell us?

The primary care team discussed the two cases as 'significant events'. At monthly significant event audit meetings the case notes of all patients with a major new diagnosis, or where care is a problem, are discussed. Such meetings offer the team insight into clinical and administrative failings.

Many primary care staff would prefer to sweep such cases under the carpet. Others fear that an open discussion of their care would result in ridicule and shame. Certainly such a discussion does require a cohesive team that is prepared to avoid finger wagging and the allocation of blame. The culture must be one in which a commitment to high-quality care is accompanied by a willingness to improve.

These two cases led to major changes in practice. Through such open discussion, team members learn how to avoid repeating mistakes and the team is able to minimise the risk of a formal complaint being lodged.

This is not an idealised vision of quality assurance. Primary care teams up and down the country already carry out significant event auditing. Later in this chapter, personal experience of the process within one team will be described. Before that, terms need to be defined and the background to significant event auditing examined.

Some definitions

Significant events are those that can be used to give an understanding of the care that an individual or team delivers. They may demonstrate good or less good care. Thus a 63-year-old man being diagnosed as having rectal carcinoma is 'significant'. In reviewing the case notes, it might become clear that best care was delivered. His family history was recorded and his higher risk was noted. When the patient presented with rectal bleeding the doctor had performed a rectal examination and referred him urgently. The hospital had responded quickly and his operation was performed within a month of presentation. He had been seen after discharge, and potential family risks and screening had been discussed with his relatives.

More often, however, at least some elements of care are found to be less than perfect. If this man had been treated with suppositories for his 'haemorrhoids' for several months before the diagnosis was made, the team could discuss the difficulties of diagnosis in rectal bleeding and how to avoid such delay in future. Although all significant events have the capacity to identify areas for improvement, most of them can also demonstrate good or appropriate care.

Some significant events are *adverse events*. These are events where something has clearly gone wrong, and the team needs to establish what happened, what was preventable and how to respond. Adverse events might therefore include, as in the two illustrative case studies above, a patient complaint, an allergic reaction to a drug which was already known about, a visit request taken but the visit not being made, a prescribing error, and so on.

A *critical incident* is a half-way house. It is an event that might indicate substandard care, but which might also occur by chance. However, the presumption is towards less good care. Any allergic reaction to a drug would be a critical incident, with the investigation aimed at establishing whether it was avoidable. Other examples of critical incidents might include an osteoporotic fracture, a stroke or a teenage pregnancy, all of which are theoretically avoidable and all of which are possible pointers to deficiencies in care.

Of the three options, it is preferable to use the term *significant event auditing*. This covers both adverse and critical events, is couched in more acceptable language, and its methodology encourages the identification and celebration of good care as well as exposure of poor care. Conceptually it is in tune with the principles of adult learning, and psychologically it is less likely to provoke a defensive response.

Behind these terms lies the concept of *risk management*[1] (*see* Chapter 11). In every consultation there is a chance that the process of care might be suboptimal. Risk management is the process by which that chance is reduced. Significant event auditing is a method for reducing clinical risk. Efficient administrative systems, a good complaints procedure, decision support, conventional auditing, error trapping (double-checking of prescriptions) and a positive culture with regard to quality are all of value in risk management.

Inevitably, all of us could do better. We can therefore use significant event auditing to gather insight for personal development. Cases can feed into educational needs and personal and practice development plans. By studying the care delivered by other members of the team, we can identify ways in which patients may be put at risk, and we can both personally and as teams work to minimise that possibility. If something has gone wrong, we can determine how to respond – often with an apology and action to ensure that it is unlikely to happen again. If the ultimate risk for health professionals is a formal complaint, significant event auditing reduces that risk. If the risk for patients is less than ideal care, the system helps to minimise this.

The background to significant event auditing

Significant event auditing is not new. Much of our core medical knowledge comes from descriptions of single cases or of a small series of cases. The links between clinical signs and pathology were established through post-mortems. A well-conducted ward round can be seen as a 'prototype significant event audit meeting', with sharing of experience and knowledge and a striving for excellence.

While primary care opted to concentrate on clinical auditing of cohorts of patients, our hospital colleagues refined the perinatal mortality meeting into the confidential enquiry into maternity deaths.[2] There is now an expanding range of such enquiries, including those into peri-operative deaths, asthma deaths,[3] suicides[4] and deaths following accidents.[5] Increasingly, these enquiries involve examining care outside hospitals as well.

When the idea of auditing 'significant events' in primary care was first published,[6,7] it appeared radical because it ran counter to the prevailing culture. However, it has become increasingly clear that it was a concept that was mould-able to meet a range of needs. One of the most widely published uses has been the examination of case records following death.[8–10]

Basically, any systematic examination of individual case records in an attempt to improve care for others can fly under this banner. For example, some practitioners have reflected on cases where patients have made complaints.[11] There is a strong belief, admittedly based on anecdote rather than on research, that openness in handling complaints, even to the extent of telling patients when they have experienced negligence, will ultimately protect the clinician.[12]

The technique has been used to explore the interval between a patient first presenting with a symptom (which in retrospect was the first sign of cancer) and action being taken,[13] the processes underlying difficult prescribing decisions[14] and the use of investigations.[15] In other countries it has been used to reflect on 'near misses' and adverse events, some of which are avoidable.[16,17]

One study used significant event auditing techniques to shed light on why signifi-cant event auditing may work.[18] A total of 100 clinicians, half of whom were GPs, were asked to discuss recent changes in their clinical practice. They reported an aver-age of three reasons per change, neatly fitting the concept of triangulation. This sug-gests that we usually change our behaviour after reinforcement from three sources. A speaker at a lunchtime seminar says that all patients with a stroke need a scan to establish whether it is a bleed or a clot. A leader in a well-respected journal says the same thing. And in a discussion about a patient who has had a stroke, the district nurse says that it is policy in the neighbouring practice to admit all strokes. Three similar messages delivered in different ways – and clinical behaviour changes as a result.

Thus significant event auditing has a long tradition, but mainly in secondary care settings. It makes use of the rich learning material in clinical records, and it can be adapted to examine any aspect of care. However, it does need a supportive team without a culture of blame. It needs a willingness to reflect and improve (as espoused by the concept of lifelong learning) and, if used effectively, it may reduce the risks of working in high-risk clinical professions.

Significant event auditing by one primary care team

One particular death in the treatment room in our practice triggered our team's interest in regular significant event auditing. Although three doctors attempted resuscitation, the patient died. In our subsequent discussions we felt that, given the size of the infarction, resuscitation was hopeless. However, we recognised a whole range of issues that we had to address. These ranged from skills in cardio-pulmonary resuscitation (CPR), through the maintenance of equipment, to the non-availability of a defibrillator.

One case, albeit a dramatic one, resulted in a wide range of changes. Over ten years ago, therefore, we started meeting every two months and, after a few meetings, monthly. We identify new cases (*see* Box 12.1) of myocardial infarction, stroke, un-planned pregnancy and cancer from the computer; acute admissions for asthma, diabetes and epilepsy are noted from hospital discharge sheets; and complaints, prescribing errors, delayed diagnoses and administrative foul-ups are picked up by all of us. Any member of the primary care team can list any case for potential consideration, and we usually have between 10 and 15 to consider every month.

Box 12.1   Potential significant events

- New cases of myocardial infarction
- New cases of stroke
- Unplanned pregnancies
- New diagnoses of malignancy
- Acute admissions for asthma, diabetes or epilepsy
- Patients' complaints
- Prescribing errors
- Delayed diagnoses
- Administrative 'foul-ups'

The meeting lasts for one hour over lunch (sandwiches are used as an incentive, although as this is the most popular of our team meetings, an incentive is probably unnecessary). The doctors, practice and community nurses and managers start by reviewing the decisions that were made at the last meeting. The team then discusses relevant patients and events, going around the room until everyone has had a chance to make a contribution.

Some discussions are very short. For example, a 16-year-old girl has had a termination of pregnancy. She had been on the contraceptive pill, and we have documented that she knew about postcoital contraception. The operation was arranged quickly and satisfactorily and she is now on the pill again. Opportunities for prevention were taken, care was good, the team is congratulated and the discussion moves on.

However, some discussions are lengthy. A 56-year-old man has come home after a myocardial infarction. Did we know about his smoking, alcohol consumption, body mass index, exercise and family history? Had we offered lifestyle advice? Does he come within the guidelines for screening for lipids? If so, was this done? Who attended the acute event and were they fully equipped? What has been done about rehabilitation?

There are four possible outcomes of these discussions, and often they occur together for the same case (*see* Box 12.2). First, and most importantly, significant event auditing can identify good practice. How often do we congratulate our colleagues on good care? For example, a patient attended the nurse for a flu vaccination. The nurse noticed that the patient was pale and a little breathless. She took a full blood count that showed a chronic leukaemia. The team recognises and congratulates her on her initiative.

Box 12.2   Outcomes from significant event auditing

- Good practice identified and acknowledged
- Further investigation carried out (e.g. literature review)
- Immediate change implemented
- No lessons to be learned – normal primary care

The second outcome is to investigate the situation further. This may take the form of obtaining advice from another doctor, undertaking a literature review, seeking out a guideline, or talking to the patient and their family. Precipitate action in response to an event may be unwise, but failure to reflect on what may have happened is equally unwise. This link between events and the educational needs of individuals and the whole team is, in our experience, very powerful.

Thirdly, we may agree that immediate change is required. For example, a doctor gave an injection on a home visit and only afterwards discovered that the drug was out of date. Fortunately, the patient has come to no harm, but clearly this cannot happen again. It is decided to institute a system for regular checking of all drugs in doctors' bags. At the next meeting the team check that the new system is in place and working.

The last outcome of our discussions is to agree that there are no lessons to be learned. The case illustrates normal primary care, and there are no particular features to be discussed in depth. These are the most common cases, but they cannot necessarily be identified in advance.

Our team is now very experienced in handling significant event audit meetings, but we have learned to abide by certain rules. Any primary care team that is setting out to undertake significant event audit would be well advised to follow the guidelines listed in Box 12.3, and the role of the chair (or external facilitator if used) is critical (*see* Box 12.4).

Box 12.3 Guidelines for significant event audit meetings

- In general, chosen cases will have had a poor outcome or a 'near miss'.
- Significant event auditing is not an appropriate technique in cases where legal action is anticipated or where individual incompetence is suspected.
- All of the members of the relevant multidisciplinary group involved in providing the care should participate.
- The aim is to be supportive to team members – all feedback should be constructive, not negative.
- It is not an attempt to search for the 'right way', but a means of exploring possible alternatives for the future.
- The chair (or external facilitator if one is used) should not have been actively involved in the case under discussion.
- A brief, anonymised, written summary of the case can be made available at the meeting, providing key dates and relevant factual information.
- The case should be introduced by a brief presentation from the involved team member(s).
- The chair should compile a written summary of the general conclusions with any actions to be taken, for review at a future specified date.
- The chair's summary should be the only record of the meeting.
- Individual team members' actions in the care of the case and their contributions to its discussion at the meeting should not be discussed outside the meeting.

Box 12.4 Role of the chair (or external facilitator if one is used)

- To explain the aims and process of the discussion.
- To structure the discussion – that is, to keep to time, to encourage contributions from all participants, and to clarify and summarise frequently.
- To maintain the basic ground rules of group discussion – for example, to allow uninterrupted discourse, to encourage participants to speak for themselves (using 'I', not 'we'), and to maintain confidentiality.
- To clarify suggestions for improvement and identify who will be responsible for initiating change.
- To recognise, acknowledge and enable appropriate expression of emotion within the group.

- To remain 'external' to the group and to avoid giving unwarranted opinions or colluding with the group during discussions.
- To compile a written summary of general conclusions with any actions to be taken, for review at a specified later date.

Adapted from Robinson LA *et al*. (1995) Use of facilitated case discussions for significant event auditing. *BMJ*. **311**: 315–18.

Conclusions

Significant event auditing encompasses a range of techniques for examining and learning from individual cases. It is a team activity and requires a mature and committed team. There is increasing evidence that, when used properly, it can be an effective catalyst for promoting quality of care and professional development. It can also help primary care teams to manage their risks, reducing the potential for things to go wrong in future. And it is clearly linked to evidence-based practice and the adoption of guidelines and best practice.

These characteristics make it an ideal feature of clinical governance. Significant event auditing can be the method at the centre of reflective practice, keeping up to date and responding to patients. However, it is not enough on its own. Just as a calorie-controlled diet needs to be combined with exercise in order to achieve weight loss, so significant event auditing works best when it is part of a quality culture applied through a range of mechanisms. For example, significant event auditing cannot replace conventional cohort auditing, but it gives it added power.

Hopefully, the last note is redundant at this point in the chapter. Most doctors and nurses in primary care are motivated by an interest in people and a desire to improve health. Significant event auditing connects them with real people in a way that a table of results in a conventional audit cannot do. That emotional content is why significant events are interesting, and why discussing them is effective. Change is an emotional process, and significant event auditing uses emotional engagement to achieve improvements in patient care and 'make them stick'.

Practical points

- Significant event auditing is a technique that provides a structured approach to case discussions.
- General lessons can be learned from individual cases.
- The term 'significant event' is preferable to 'critical' or 'adverse' event, and covers both.
- Significant event auditing is an effective means of reducing clinical risk and promoting quality of care and professional development.
- It requires a mature and committed team with a supportive, reflective and 'no-blame' culture.

References

1 Vincent C (1997) Risk, safety, and the dark side of quality. *BMJ*. **314**: 1775–6.
2 Hibbard B and Milner D (1994) Reports on confidential enquiries into maternal deaths: an audit of previous recommendations. *Health Trends*. **26**: 26–8.
3 Mohan G, Harrison B, Badminton R, Mildenhall S and Wareham N (1996) A confidential enquiry into deaths caused by asthma in an English health region: implications for general practice. *Br J Gen Pract*. **46**: 529–32.
4 Matthews K, Milne S and Ashcroft G (1994) Role of doctors in the prevention of suicide: the final consultation. *Br J Gen Pract*. **44**: 345–8.
5 Hussain L and Redmond A (1994) Are pre-hospital deaths from accidental injury preventable? *BMJ*. **308**: 1077–80.
6 Pringle M, Bradley C, Carmichael C, Wallis H and Moore A (1995) *Significant Event Auditing*. Occasional Paper 70. Royal College of General Practitioners, London.
7 Pringle M and Bradley C (1994) Significant event auditing: a user's guide. *Audit Trends*. **2**: 20–3.
8 Robinson L, Stacy R, Spencer J and Bhopal R (1995) Use of facilitated case discussions for significant event auditing. *BMJ*. **311**: 315–18.
9 Khunti K (1996) A method of creating a death register for general practice. *BMJ*. **312**: 952.
10 Holden J, O'Donnell S, Brindley J and Miles L (1998) Analysis of 1263 deaths in four general practices. *Br J Gen Pract*. **48**: 1409–12.
11 Pietroni R and de Uray-Ura S (1994) Informal complaints procedure in general practice: first year's experience. *BMJ*. **308**: 1546–8.
12 Ritchie J and Davies S (1995) Professional negligence: a duty of candid disclosure? *BMJ*. **310**: 888–9.
13 Holden J and Pringle M (1995) Delay pattern analysis of 446 patients in nine practices. *Audit Trends*. **3**: 96–8.
14 Bradley C and Riaz A (1998) Barriers to effective asthma care in inner-city general practice. *Eur J Gen Pract*. **4**: 65–8.
15 Robling M, Kinnersley P, Houston H, Hourihan M, Cohen D and Hale J (1998) An exploration of GPs' use of MRI: a critical incident study. *Fam Pract*. **15**: 236–43.
16 Britt H, Miller G, Steven I *et al.* (1997) Collecting data on potentially harmful events: a method for monitoring incidents in general practice. *Fam Pract*. **14**: 101–6.
17 Bhasale A (1998) The wrong diagnosis: identifying causes of potentially adverse events in general practice using incident monitoring. *Fam Pract*. **15**: 308–18.
18 Allery L, Owen P and Robling M (1997) Why general practitioners and consultants change their clinical practice: a critical incident study. *BMJ*. **314**: 870–4.

CHAPTER 13

Lessons from complaints

Arthur Bullough and Ruth Etchells

When people cease to complain, they cease to think.

Napoleon I

> This chapter explores current complaints procedures which mainly affect general practitioners, and offers lessons that can be learned from complainants both locally and in the wider NHS.

The context: current complaint structures and their history

Complaints procedures: necessary (resented) evil or ineffective good?

Few aspects of the NHS arouse stronger feelings in both clinicians and patients than the issue of appropriate complaints procedures. All sides accept that mechanisms must exist for handling patient dissatisfaction efficiently and effectively. After all, the NHS should be accountable to the public. Yet many GPs would also ruefully argue that the same need exists for handling their own complaints against patients.

- A working definition of a complaint is 'any expression of dissatisfaction that needs a response'.
- Information from complaints is free feedback about your service. This is the best form of market research you can get.

From *How to Deal with Complaints*, Cabinet Office

Both public services and commercial organisations recognise that handling complaints *well* can bring immense benefits, and this is perhaps the first and most important lesson to learn from complaints. They make available important information about the current style of practice in a particular locality or practice. If used positively, a good complaints procedure can help individual doctors, the whole practice team or even a whole health organisation not only to avoid similar situations elsewhere but also to improve services generally. At the very least, it can save time and resources which would otherwise be spent on protracted disputes, and it *should* lead to improvement in practitioner–patient relationships across the board.

'Necessary evil?'

'Should' … Ay, there's the rub. For it has to be faced that there remains (although far less sharply than with the pre-1996 process) a dichotomy between GPs' perceptions of the complaints process and that of the public in general, and complainants in particular. Many GPs and primary care teams are hard-pressed by a variety of administrative and legislative demands – needing to keep up with the fast-moving pace of developing medical research, pushed to meet the ever-increasing demands of patients and wanting to effect preventive medicine, but lacking the resources in time or staff to do so. To find themselves the target of a complaint is to feel themselves unjustly put on trial, however informal the process. Thus to many the Government-imposed complaints procedure may indeed be 'necessary', but feel 'evil', in that even if it does not go on to the now rare formal disciplinary hearing, it can be perceived as unfair or even threatening, and can cause much stress.

Case 1

Complainant Z reported that there had been no acknowledgement of a complaint, made in writing to the GP concerned, about the medical care offered to a spouse during what proved to be a terminal illness. Dr A, when contacted about this, stated that he had received no such letter. A second copy was sent, which was also copied to the health authority, from which it was apparent that the complaint lacked serious substance. When nothing had been heard from Dr A by either the complainant or the health authority, the latter contacted him in order to offer reassurance and help, only to hear with dismay that Dr A had felt so stressed on receiving the complaint that he had felt it made his professional life unendurable, and he had that very day resigned from the practice.

'Ineffective good?'

Conversely, complainants feel that they are at a disadvantage when making a complaint. They often show an ambivalent attitude towards their GP. This arises partly from a widespread sense of inequality with their doctor, who is often much better educated, more articulate and more socially confident than they are. Their doctor is in some sense their 'judge' whenever they ask for clinical help. The relationship often starts to go wrong when the patient feels that the *manner* of the GP towards them is abrupt, dismissive or demeaning. At the same time, it is clear from the tenor of many of the complaints we have processed that patient expectations of the medical profession have increased, and in many cases are unrealistic – and sometimes wholly unreasonable.

The GP is (still) assumed by many to be properly available 24 hours a day, however minor the case. There is a more deeply held assumption, unexamined but clearly evident in many of the cases we have explored, that if only the GP was 'doing the job properly', the patient would not have suffered as he or she did, would have recovered more quickly and more fully, would not have died, and so on. Add to this cocktail of social anxiety and clinical expectation the emotions of bereavement (grief and anger, and even unexplored guilt, which complainants sometimes bring to the process) and it will be obvious why the procedure sometimes seems to the complainants like a 'good' which does not deliver the goods. To them it is 'ineffective' because it could never in fact meet such a complex set of needs.

Against this background of strongly contrasted needs, hopes and fears of the GP on the one hand and the complainant on the other, the Government reassessed what a complaints process should attempt to achieve, and what it could not, and how complaints might be better processed – more effectively, less stressfully and more quickly. Behind any attempt to set up a more effective complaints procedure there are contrasting principles, and we need to be aware of what these are in the present system.

New approach needed?

The present complaints procedure, which the Government brought into effect in April 1996, after much taking of evidence, was based on two major principles which differed sharply from what had gone before. First and most fundamental was the separation of complaints from disciplinary procedures. *A complaint sustained no longer implies breach of contract.* This clearly rejects the principle (tacitly held by some members of the general public and assumed by GPs) that a complaints procedure must in some sense be punitive in its intention. So long as this notion pervaded the process, it was inevitable that GPs would be thrown on the defensive and would find it difficult to engage whole-heartedly in co-operative discernment. Yet this is what effective complaints procedures really require.

Moreover, because of the quasi-judicial nature of the proceedings under the previous system, it was difficult for doctors to make any kind of personal apology for something that with hindsight could have been handled better. Often an apology was all that was actually required. It would have restored some kind of dignity to the doctor–patient relationship, and offered recognition that all had not been done (or said) well, and that this had caused the complainant (or the patient on whose behalf the complainant spoke) unnecessary distress.

Local resolution: 'owning' the process

The second major change was that complaints should always be dealt with informally, in the first instance, at practice level. The two governing principles here, both of which are new to the process, are subsidiarity and informality. The procedures are therefore much more immediate and accessible, inviting a combined effort from doctor and complainant, both of whom are invited to 'own' the process in an attempt to resolve the issue (*see* Box 13.1). This is co-operative discernment. Where this is not successful, other strategies – including informal conciliation – are offered by the local primary care trust. Only in the rarest cases should the matter go before a formal review panel.

Box 13.1   The key objectives of the 'local resolution process'

- Ease of access for patients and complainants
- A simplified procedure
- Separation of complaints from disciplinary procedures
- Making use of information from complaints to improve services
- Fairness to staff and complainants alike
- A more rapid, open process
- The primary aim of resolving the problem and satisfying the concerns of the complainant

---

The present complaints procedure: the structure

A diagram of the current complaints procedure is shown in Figure 13.1.

Since 1996, all practices have been required to have an in-house complaints procedure, the details of which must be clearly publicised to their patients. They must:

- appoint a complaints manager and also an overseeing GP for clinical complaints
- draw up a complaints code of practice and ensure that staff follow it
- display a notice about the practice's complaints procedure and have leaflets available at reception.

Local resolution process, stage 1: complaints to practice

1 What about?

Anything! Premises, administration, delays and manner of reception, as well as clinical issues, are all legitimate material for complaint if they are felt to be less than satisfactory, since each is part of the total service offered. Sometimes a non-clinical matter is actually revealing some quite serious difficulty within the practice itself.

Case 2

Complainant Y wrote to complain that the services being provided by Dr B had deteriorated significantly. The doctor was said to be spending less time with his patients, the practice premises were not being maintained to acceptable standards, and practice staff were not being treated in an acceptable manner.

When this complaint was followed up, it became clear that what could appear initially to be general apathy on the part of the doctor in fact went far deeper. It was established that the reason for many of the problems was that Dr B was in dispute with a fellow GP who shared the premises. Many bills for which the doctors had shared responsibilities, including gas and electricity, had not been settled.

What had begun as a complaint about a deterioration in service provision had revealed a serious professional problem in the relationship between two GPs, which was undoubtedly having consequences for the services that they offered.

On regular occasions the receipt of a complaint against a contractor can be indicative of other problems within a practice.

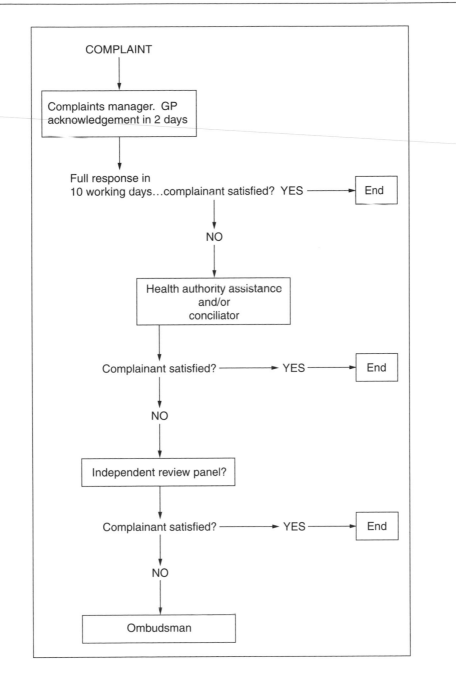

Figure 13.1   The complaints procedure.

2 Who by?
   Patients or former patients of a practitioner. Complaints may also be made on
   behalf of existing or former patients by anyone who has the patient's consent.
3 When?
   Normally within six months of an incident occurring or within 12 months of it
   coming to light. Discretionary extension is possible depending on the circumstances.

4 What happens?
- Complaints are made to the practice, orally or in writing, and are dealt with by whatever process the practice has set up.
- An acknowledgement or initial response must normally be made by the practice within two working days.
- An explanation or more detailed response must normally be provided within 10 working days.
- A careful record must be kept.
- At the conclusion of all discussions the practice must send a letter to the complainant summarising all investigation, action and discussion which has followed the complaint.
5 And if the complainant is not satisfied?
Sometimes the primary care trust complaints manager can, with the consent of both parties, act as an 'honest broker' between the GP and the complainant in order to move the matter towards resolution. Indeed, if this is requested, such an intervention can take place at the earliest stage. This is particularly important if the complainant has no confidence in the practice's complaints procedures, or if there is a strong personality clash. The resolution would still be taking place 'in-house', with the primary care trust merely acting as a facilitator of the negotiations at practice level.

Should the above procedure fail, there is a further possibility.

Local resolution process, stage 2: conciliation process

Each primary care trust has a number of trained conciliators available who can offer assistance whenever a practice or a complainant requests it. Their task is to facilitate agreement, and their work is therefore treated as wholly confidential. They must never be required to report in detail to primary care trusts on the details of cases in which they are involved. Their role is most effective when they are used as early as possible to resolve complaints. Practices would be wise to draw upon their expertise without delay if it seems that the complainant is resistant to or dissatisfied with the practice's first attempt at resolution, even if the practice has been assisted by primary care trust personnel.

It is recognised that the normal time target of 10 working days to provide a full response to a complaint may need an extension if the services of a conciliator are deemed to be necessary.

If the matter still remains unresolved even after the intervention of a conciliator, there is a further option for the complainant.

Stage 3: independent review panel

Complainants who remain dissatisfied after the local resolution process can ask the primary care trust convenor (either orally or in writing) for an independent review panel. The request has to be made within a given time limit.

It is the local convenor (appointed by the primary care trust) who must decide whether an independent review panel is appropriate. The right to request one does not carry with it automatic consent. The convenor will always inform the GP of the request, and will ask for a copy of the exchange of correspondence to date, together with the records kept by the practice of the whole process. The complainant must submit a letter setting out their remaining grievances and why they are dissatisfied with the outcome of the local resolution process. The convenor must then, in consultation with an independent lay chairman appointed from a list approved by the Secretary of State for Health – and, where clinical issues are involved, an independent medical adviser – decide whether:

- the GP or practice team can take any further action to satisfy the complainant
- the practice has already taken all practical action and establishing a panel would add no further value to the process.

In the light of these decisions the convenor will either agree to set up a panel or not. Both the complainant and the doctor are advised of the decision and the reasons for it.

The chief objective of the panel is to resolve the grievance in a conciliatory manner, and it *may not make any suggestion in its report that anyone should be subject to disciplinary action*. To this conciliatory end it may determine for itself its method, choosing a style that is appropriate to the particular circumstances, and on no account allowing a confrontational situation to arise. For instance, the panel (of three members) together with clinical advice of at least two doctors nominated by their professional bodies may meet with the complainant and the doctor separately, or it may decide upon smaller meetings with only one member of the panel present to meet the two parties (although always with an assessor if a clinical matter is in debate).

The assessors will report in writing to the panel, which will normally attach such reports to its own final report, after checking a draft with the doctor and complainant to ensure factual accuracy.

The GP, complainant and anyone else who has been interviewed by the panel next receive a copy of the final report. Where appropriate, the doctor may need to show parts of the report to colleagues in the practice, while recognising its confidential nature. The primary care trust chief executive and chairman also receive a copy of the report, and the chief executive will write to the complainant about any action that the primary care trust is taking as a result of the panel's work.

At the same time, the complainant will be reminded that there remains a further stage if they remain dissatisfied.

Stage 4: the ombudsman
Reference may only be made to the ombudsman when the NHS processes have been exhausted. Therefore, the complainant may only move on to this stage if they are either:

- refused an independent review panel

or

- dissatisfied with the work of the independent review panel that has been set up at their request.

Lessons from complaints

Some statistics regarding complaints made in County Durham are shown in Boxes 13.2 and 13.3.

Box 13.2 Statistics 1997–98 for County Durham

Total number of written complaints against general medical practitioners	585
Number of such complaints resolved by practice	557
Number of such complaints resolved following assistance from health authority and/or conciliator	16
Number of applications for independent review	8
Number of independent review applications granted	3
Number of cases referred to ombudsman	1

Box 13.3 Types of complaint 1997–98 for County Durham

Communication/attitude of the general practitioner	30%
Clinical	28%
Anciliary staff/premises/other	21%
Practice management	18%
Administration	3%
Receptionists/other staff	2%
Removal of patient from list	2%

What complainants want

There is a view that the majority of people who complain about their experiences of the NHS are seeking financial compensation. However, studies have found that this is not so. Compensation is by no means the most popular motive. In fact complainants want:

- acknowledgement of the incident
- an explanation in clear lay language
- an apology
- reassurance that preventive action will be taken to ensure that there is no repetition of the incident.

More rarely people shift from wanting the GP to be accountable to wanting consequent punishment. Compensation seekers also belong to this smaller group – indeed, to some extent they coincide. In our experience, fewer than 1% of complainants make it explicit that they are seeking financial compensation.

How to use a complaint positively

The most important lesson concerns attitude. It has emerged quite clearly from experience of complaints processes that where doctors and other staff are receptive to complaints, and see them not as personal assaults but as useful information – indicators of a public perception and of possible improvement of services – really fruitful results can ensue.

For the individual, positive reactions would include the following:

- acknowledging the complaint quickly, and always thanking complainants for bringing matters to the practice's attention
- sharing the matter with someone – a colleague, the local medical committee (LMC), practice manager, defence organisation and/or primary care trust complaints manager (who has a wealth of experience and can often help to sort out matters quickly)
- working with the local community health council, to whom the complainant will often turn for advice and representation, remembering that resolution of a complaint is a co-operative effort. (Community Health Councils were abolished in December 2003. Independent Complaints Advisory Services are being established in their place)
- although meeting the 10-day deadline for a full response after investigation, also taking time before drafting the response (this gives an opportunity for the first shock, and possibly anger, to be replaced by a calmer and more thoughtful approach, a tone that is more likely to engage with the complainant, and a thorough investigation and assembly of relevant documents)
- offering a meeting with the complainant, *but only if both complainant and practitioner* genuinely want this, and the meeting has a clear purpose (disputing fact is rarely useful)
- writing a full response which is informative, truthful and expressed in a language that will be understood. Some clinical terminology can have a radically different meaning for a lay person, and such misunderstandings can trigger or compound a complaint
- being prepared to say 'sorry'. If after investigation it seems that the standard of care was lower than it should have been, an apology should be made. Our experience is that the word 'sorry' is the most useful tool when handling complaints. *Note*: Many general practitioners fear that they will admit liability if they apologise. It is for this reason, among others, that 'accountability' has been separated from 'liability' in the complaints process. The Medical Defence Union comments that a detailed explanation should always be given in response to complaints, and also an apology if it is recognised as appropriate. However, this does *not* constitute an admission of liability.

For a practice team, positive reactions would include the following:

- taking corporate responsibility for complaints, with each team member giving support and encouragement to any member who is faced with a complaint. Our experience is that this is not always the case. The resolution of the complaint can then be more difficult, the doctor more distressed and the practice itself less effective
- taking any action that is found to be necessary to prevent repetition of the incident, outlining in their response their proposed remedies. It is unwise to guarantee that the incident will not recur, but sensible to guarantee that the situation will be kept under review.

Case 3

Complainant X's case concerned his wife, for whom the diagnosis of cancer of the stomach and liver had been in his view unreasonably slow, pre-empting effective intervention, due to what were perceived to be inappropriate delays in referral on the part of the two GPs involved, Drs C and D. The history of the disease (as noted) began with visits to the surgery in January, February and March, with the patient complaining of 'wind', dyspepsia and steady weight loss. Dr C's working diagnosis in March was of peptic ulcer or gall-stones, although in view of the weight loss, she thought a malignancy was possible. A blood test was arranged, but was not attended by the patient because of family commitments (her daughter had had a baby).

By April, new symptoms of cough (in a smoker) offered to Dr D prompted him to make a tentative diagnosis of lung cancer. Under pressure, the patient attended a blood test (which proved normal) and a chest X-ray was urgently arranged, which also proved normal. This prompted Dr C to review her working diagnosis to one of upper gastrointestinal malignancy. After further blood and urine samples had been taken (which also proved normal), she wrote to a consultant asking for an urgent appointment for the patient for assessment and further examination. Both Drs C and D were unaware that there would be a four-week delay.

It was not therefore until the beginning of July that the patient had a hospital appointment, and not until 1 August that an endoscopy was available. This and a CT scan performed two days later indicated an extensive gastric tumour, with further 'likely deposits' in the liver. No treatment was appropriate, and the patient died in November.

Lessons for wider reference in the NHS

The primary care trust monitors all complaints (*see* Box 13.2) and takes note of any issues particular to the practice which may have wider implications for primary care in general (Case 3 above is a case in point). Most primary care trusts arrange training sessions on complaints so that primary care team members can draw on what colleagues have learned from their experience of complaints. Practices are well advised to send a representative to these events.

Practices are also requested to undertake regular audits of patient complaints, and to explain how these have been processed using in-house procedures. To widen the scope, complaints that have been resolved immediately within the practice can be compared with those where conciliation or independent review was necessary. Practice guidelines can be developed and modified as a result, and outcomes fed back to the primary care trusts on the one hand and the LMC on the other.

Many LMCs ask the primary care trusts to keep them informed of issues raised through the complaints procedure.

Future improvements to the Complaints Procedure

In March 2003 the Department of Health issued a document entitled *NHS Complaints Reform: making things right*.

This document sets out the Government's plans to improve the NHS complaints procedure following:

- an independent two-year evaluation of the complaints procedure, and
- a listening exercise to gather feedback in relation to suggestions made by a team of researchers.

It sets out a comprehensive programme for reform, elements of which will be subject to primary legislation.

The planned changes build on the existing procedures and will introduce operational improvements, including the following:

- the need to improve support for people who are making a complaint
- better communication and customer-care training for those involved in dealing with complaints
- NHS organisations to be held accountable for the performance of complaints handling
- reform of the Independent Review Panels process by placing responsibility with the Commission for Healthcare Audit and Inspection, the intention being that those who remain dissatisfied with the response they have received from the local resolution process have access to a neutral and impartial view of their case.

And finally

Co-operative discernment of why things may have gone wrong, and how they can be improved, is not a bad basis for learning from complaints.

Further reading

- Department of Health (1994) *Being Heard: the report of a review committee on NHS procedures*. HMSO, London.
- NHS Executive (1996) *Practice-Based Conflicts Procedure: guidance for general practices*. HMSO, London.
- Department of Health (2003) *NHS Complaints Reform: making things right*. Department of Health, London.

Practical points

- Handling complaints well brings benefits.
- Good complaints procedures provide free information about the practice.
- Protracted disputes cost time and money, and are very stressful to all concerned.
- Some practitioners take complaints too much to heart.
- Both practices and patients feel at a disadvantage within the complaints system.
- The complaints process separates complaints from disciplinary procedures.
- Often an apology by the practitioner is all that is needed.
- All practices must now appoint a complaints manager and an overseeing GP, have a complaints code of practice, and advertise the fact.
- Non-clinical complaints can reveal quite serious difficulties within a practice.
- Most complainants want reassurance that, if at all possible, the incident will not happen again.

CHAPTER 14

Tackling poor performance

George Taylor

We are what we repeatedly do; excellence, then, is not an act but a habit.

Aristotle

> This chapter highlights how poor clinical performance is now everyone's business, something that can no longer be ignored or quietly tolerated, and describes how better performance can be encouraged.

The individual doctor

Personal implications of clinical governance

Although clinical governance is a recently invented concept, first described in the Government White Paper *A First-Class Service: quality in the new NHS*,[1] its actual components are not new. Medical audit, a major tool of clinical governance, is now a well-established practice in medicine – a skill that is felt to be so important that it constitutes one of the components of the summative (end-point) assessment of GP vocational training. Audit allows practitioners to look at current practice and identify areas where both change and development are needed. Sometimes audit can be used to reassure practitioners that what they are doing is of an adequate or even high standard. However, some practitioners have a very narrow view of audit. They feel that it can only be true audit if figures are involved. They forget that a very valuable type of audit involves looking at significant events, where members of a multidisciplinary team can learn valuable lessons together.[2]

Other components of clinical governance include the practice of keeping up to date, aspiring to high standards, reflecting on one's work, recognising and learning from less than optimal practice, and minimising risk to patients. These are all components of traditional professionalism, and as such should hold no fears for any practitioner. What clinical governance modifies for the involved professionals is that it adds into the equation the NHS as the 'employer'. NHS involvement now demands that doctors be explicit about their activities. In the past, it was the norm for them to accept as implicit that this was what any 'good' professional did, and thus did not require monitoring. How times have changed. In 1993, the new professional role of doctors in the twenty-first century was made explicit by Donald

Irvine, then President of the General Medical Council (GMC).[3] The basic values that doctors must espouse in their daily work has been encapsulated in the GMC document *Duties of a Doctor* (*see* Box 14.1).

Box 14.1 The duties of a doctor (General Medical Council)

- Make the care of your patient your first concern.
- Treat every patient politely and considerately.
- Respect patients' dignity and privacy.
- Listen to patients and respect their views.
- Give patients information in a form that they can understand.
- Respect the right of patients to be fully involved in decisions about their care.
- Keep your professional knowledge and skills up to date.
- Recognise the limits of your professional competence.
- Be honest and trustworthy.
- Respect and protect confidential information.
- Make sure that your personal beliefs do not prejudice your patient's care.
- Act quickly to protect the patient from risk if you believe that you or a colleague may not be fit to practise.
- Avoid abusing your position as a doctor.
- Work with colleagues in the ways that best serve patients' interests.

The individual and the practice: maintaining good performance

Until recently, much education in primary care has been unplanned and unstructured. Here individual professionals attend educational events – often a lecture by a local hospital expert, usually away from the workplace, and driven by personal wants rather than identified educational needs.[4] Some practices organise regular educational meetings in the workplace, ranging from useful team activities (e.g. discussing team roles in the management of a chronic disease) to a meeting sponsored by a pharmaceutical company ('drug lunch'). The latter type of meeting may well have social value and also be of marketing value to the company involved, but often seems to lack educational content. In contrast, informal learning takes place in the course of every working day, but frequently is not recognised as the potent source of education that it actually is. Activities such as learning about drugs or patient management from specialists' letters, using information sources such as books or the computer during consultations, and just talking with colleagues about problems, are all activities that take place in every surgery, yet are often under-valued educationally. This low educational status has been reinforced by NHS regulations covering the continuing education of general practitioners. The Post-graduate Education Allowance (PGEA) regulations[5] value formal meetings as sources of postgraduate education allowance credits, yet make it difficult for personal learning of an informal nature to be recognised. The underlying philosophy seems to be driven by the belief, encapsulated in the writing of McGregor,[6] that people will avoid doing their best if they can. In reality, one should recognise that the vast majority of people want to do a good job.

The Chief Medical Officer's review[7] proposed that continuing education should be based on a personal educational plan (PEP). These plans were to be developed using tools for the assessment of educational need, alongside simple evaluations which could measure progress or identify when progress was not being made. The CMO's report also suggested that educational planning could be a whole-practice activity, leading to the production of a practice professional development plan (PPDP). The major change suggested by both of these proposals was that individuals could tailor their education not only to meet their personal wants, but also to fulfil their individually identified needs. Moreover, it went further, recognising that professionals had a responsibility not only to themselves, but also to the practice, the locality and the NHS, when planning their education.

If they took these changes on board, practices would be developing education within the practice as a team activity. They would be recognising the value of education to their team by giving protected time during the working day for practitioners to investigate and learn about areas of benefit to the practice. Study leave to go elsewhere to learn skills to benefit the team would become the norm, rather than an episodic finding. The use of critical incident audits (involving the whole team) would enable the practice to learn together both from their successes and from what had not gone well. At the very minimum, this type of learning would improve teamworking,[8] and it seems likely that it would also improve standards of care.

Causes of poor performance

What, then, are the implications of these educational developments in relation to issues of performance? We know that doctors often develop difficulties with performance over a period of many years with a gradual slide into poor performance, possibly as a result of their not keeping up to date, and this not being recognised and remedial action taken. The doctor may be unaware of the problem, and in the past other team members and colleagues may not have felt that it was their place to discuss it with him or her. However, if practitioners are engaged in both practice and personal needs assessment exercises, and are meeting for developmental activity and learning, concerns should be identified at an early stage, when major loss of face is not an issue. One might postulate that this would lead to early remedial education before any such problems became significant enough to have an effect on patient care.

Doctors working alone may experience more difficulty, as they do not have working colleagues to 'bounce things off'. They must not be diffident about using the local educational network of GP tutors or primary care trust educationalists to help them in this task.

In 2002, a further initiative to help doctors to identify needs at an early stage was introduced, namely GP appraisal. Primary care trusts must now ensure that their GPs have annual appraisal.[9] There were early fears that this was an ill-thought-out Government initiative aimed at identifying, naming and shaming 'bad' doctors. If appraisal is to be effective, it must be developmental and essentially kept confidential between the appraiser and the person being appraised.[10] Thankfully this seems to be the direction in which appraisal is now developing. Annual appraisal is now linked to GMC revalidation, the introduction of which has been repeatedly delayed. Revalidation should also therefore be a spur to personal review and maintenance of good performance.[11]

Other factors that may cause poor performance

It is easy to fall into the trap of believing that education is the only factor to consider when performance is poor, and that the answer to any performance problem is 'a course' or a period of retraining. International experience[12] makes it clear that factors such as physical and mental health, alcohol and drug abuse, working conditions and isolation from other practitioners are all frequently involved. It was only recently that the theoretical provision of occupational health services for GPs was proposed,[13] and at the time of writing, provision across the UK is still patchy. Historically, organisations such as the British Medical Association local medical committees (LMCs) set up support services for practitioners. The uptake of these services was usually low,[14] possibly because of the traditional GP value of coping and 'getting on with it'. The 'new doctor' in the twenty-first century seems less likely to put their health at risk, more likely to use services such as confidential counselling, and more aware of the new professionalism that is developing within general practice (see Box 14.2). Yorkshire has had a system of confidential educational mentors for some years. Uptake in the past has been low, but younger doctors are now seeking out and using this service.[15]

Box 14.2   Features of the twenty-first-century doctor (after Irvine[3])

- Clear professional values
- Explicit standards
- Collective as well as personal responsibility for standards of practice
- Local medical regulation based on teams
- Systematic evidence of keeping up to date and of adequate performance
- Effective systems for dealing with dysfunctional doctors

Equally, it is an almost impossible task to provide adequate care if you are working in a substandard building or have a significant shortage of staff or a complex and increasing workload. The answer in these situations can never be 'education'. It often requires primary care trust action, rather than action by the individual practitioner, to improve working conditions or staffing levels.

The bad

There is a small group of practitioners who are quite simply wicked and beyond help. Appraisal or revalidation of doctors would not have identified Harold

Shipman. He may even have come out as a 'committed hard-working GP' with a high home visiting rate, with visits initiated by him rather than only at the request of patients. His problem was not one that related to his profession or professionalism in general – it was simply that he was a mass murderer, and no amount of retraining would have changed him.

Performance and the health service: dealing with poor performance

Primary care trusts

In 2002, primary care trusts took over what had previously been a health authority responsibility, namely dealing with performance problems. The mechanisms that had been developed by health authorities had often used the model proposed by the Sheffield University School of Health and Related Research (SHaRR).[16] This model envisaged that most problems could and should be investigated and dealt with at a local level. SHaRR provided guidance about who should be involved in a locality, how the process should take place and how to deal with outcomes. Most local investigation should involve a senior manager, the LMC, an educationalist and sometimes lay representation. This local team would do its utmost to engage the doctor, and would try to be non-threatening. Its role would be to collect and review evidence. Only where problems appeared to be serious, repetitious and substantiated would further investigation be considered. Primary care trust teams would usually visit the practitioner and his or her colleagues to discuss the perceived problem or problems. Increasingly, an initial occupational health assessment has been advised if health is thought to be an issue. A method of assessing knowledge and skills is useful, as is observing the actual practice of the doctor if possible. This also allows an assessment of working conditions to be made. Most primary care trusts have a second group of professionals whose role is to consider the outcome of such assessments and decide on the way forward.

The Royal College of General Practitioners Quality Unit has helpfully developed a 'toolkit' for dealing with practitioners whose performance gives cause for concern. This was in response to the perceived need for more robust and explicit performance assessment mechanisms in general practice, and the relative lack of experience of many individuals involved in this activity. This 'toolkit' is available both on the Internet (www.rcgp.org.uk) and in paper format, and provides easy access to information about the management of performance problems.

Many lesser problems can be dealt with at a local level, with input from local educationalists whose role is to advise on educational solutions. However, some problems are complex and difficult to unravel. In these cases, postgraduate deaneries may be able to provide an independent local educational assessment in more depth than that usually provided by the primary care trust mechanisms. In some cases this will avoid the need for a referral to a national body.[17] For example, Yorkshire Deanery assessments are closely modelled on the National Clinical Assessment Authority's methodology (*see* below). In this way it is hoped that it will be possible to provide an educational prescription that will help the doctor to overcome his or her problems and return to competent practice. Such assessments will also be able to indicate whether educational need is a major reason for the performance problems, or whether there are other factors that the primary care trust must consider and deal with, such as the practitioner's health or their working conditions.

National Clinical Assessment Authority

In 2001, the National Clinical Assessment Authority (NCAA) was established as a special health authority,[17] as part of NHS reorganisation with the aim of improving the standards and quality of the health service. The NCAA should become involved not when a primary care trust believes that a doctor is unfit to practise, but rather when it is expected that performance issues can be identified and that a possible solution or solutions can be defined. It has a network of advisers based around the country who are available to give advice. These advisers are either experienced clinicians or health service managers. Advisers see their role as supporting primary care trusts by providing advice and ensuring that local assessments take place. They should be contacted in cases where doctors refuse to be involved in local assessment, or if the remedies that were thought to be likely to work locally have been unsuccessful. In some cases the situation will just seem too complex for primary care trust mechanisms to sort out. This identification process may be possible at a local level, and advice on how to progress may be the NCAA's role. Sometimes, however, an NCAA assessment is required. Whoever carries out the assessment, the involved primary care trust still retains responsibility, and all findings and recommendations are fed back to them for consideration and implementation. It is important to recognise that the NCAA is acting in a formative way, being educational and developmental, and is not offering a pass/fail test of fitness to practise. This is the role of the General Medical Council (*see* below). The NCAA envisages part of its future role as training primary care trust assessors (often in collaboration with postgraduate deaneries) and ensuring the common use of national instruments. Problems in Sunderland should be treated in a similar way to those in Southampton. In the past, the NHS tribunal was a theoretical route whereby a GP might be suspended and investigated. Suspension was otherwise impossible because of the GP's self-employed status. Sadly, the NHS tribunal did not work effectively, and the Health and Social Care Act (2001) abolished this body. It also introduced the power for primary care trusts to suspend GPs. Primary care trusts were also charged at this time to develop a supplementary list of locums and non-principals in their area. These doctors had been difficult to identify and track prior to 2001, and this made investigation of problems more difficult.

General Medical Council

Certain performance concerns – at whatever stage of the process, whether local, deanery or NCAA level, or coming to light as an acute new problem – demand direct referral to the General Medical Council. Because of the serious nature of these concerns, patient care may be significantly threatened and the doctor may not be fit to practise. *Duties of a Doctor* demands that in these situations the GMC must be involved. This is a major responsibility for those dealing with such cases.

GMC procedures can seem complex and time consuming.[18] All complaints are screened to identify whether they should be considered as a performance problem, a health problem or one relating to conduct. If it is felt that there may be a case to answer relating to performance, the involved doctor will be offered an assessment, and will only go straight to a hearing if they refuse this. GMC assessment reviews the doctor's experience and training and their type of daily work. This is to ensure that they are assessed by people who understand what their daily work involves. The assessment team also has lay membership. After the assessment, the team may recommend some remedial activity. If the doctor is willing to carry this out they need never attend a hearing. However, if serious factors are discovered, a formal hearing will take place.

If retraining needs are identified, the local director of postgraduate GP education is contacted and asked to consider whether the suggested retraining is possible. Some referrals from the GMC have such major recommendations that it seems likely that the only answer is to start basic medical education all over again. A clear outline of GMC procedures is available on their website (www.gmc-uk.org).

Other team members

Performance problems may sometimes be identified in other members of the team. However, doctors cannot avoid these as 'someone else's problem' – they must always uphold the 'duties of a doctor'. These other professionals are invariably salaried and will have clearly documented pathways for dealing with concerns. If doctors are uncertain how to proceed, they should contact their clinical governance lead at the primary care trust or their medical protection organisation.

Conclusion

Changes in doctors' relationships with the NHS have taken place in recent years. Professional values have developed and have been modified by the world we now inhabit. Doctors have to be more explicit about their work and about how they are keeping up to date. They can no longer give colleagues the benefit of the doubt – they have a duty to act if suboptimal practice is identified.

The development of clinical governance, and the recognition that education must not only meet personal wants but also involve the needs of the service, should lead to many performance problems being identified at an early stage. In those situations where this does not happen, clear mechanisms have developed to allow problems to be addressed at a local level. Complex situations can be investigated by the NCAA or the postgraduate deanery. In a small number of cases, the GMC performance procedures will need to be invoked.

Practical points

- It is the duty of all professionals to ensure that their clinical practice is up to date and competent.
- Professionals working in teams have a common responsibility to ensure that all team members perform satisfactorily.
- It is no longer acceptable to ignore poor performance in oneself or in others.
- Doctors are guided by the GMC's *Duties of a Doctor*.[4]
- Both formal and informal educational activities play a part in supporting good practice.
- Primary care trusts are responsible for investigating poor performance.
- Primary care trusts now have the power to suspend a doctor whose performance is giving cause for concern.
- The NCAA and GMC are national bodies that are engaged in performance issues.

References

1 NHS Executive (1998) *A First-Class Service: quality in the new NHS*. NHS Executive, Leeds.

2 Pringle M, Bradley C, Carmichael C *et al.* (1995) *Significant Event Auditing: a study of the feasibility and potential of case-based auditing in primary medical care*. Royal College of General Practitioners, London.

3 Irvine D (1999) The performance of doctors: the new professionalism. *Lancet*. **353**: 1174–7.

4 Pitts J and White P (1994) Learning objectives in general practice. Identification of wants and needs. *Educ Gen Pract*. **5**(1): 59–66.

5 NHS Executive (2000) *Statement of Fees and Allowances in General Practice*. NHS Executive, Leeds.

6 McGregor D (1990) *The Human Side of Enterprise*. McGraw Hill, New York.

7 Chief Medical Officer (1998) *A Review of Continuing Professional Development in General Practice*. Department of Health, London.

8 Pearson P and Spencer J (eds) (1997) Outcome measures for teamwork in primary care. In: *Promoting Teamwork in Primary Care*. Arnold, London.

9 www.doh.gov.uk/gpappraisal (accessed 5 November 2002).

10 Jelley D (2001) *Appraisal in General Practice in the Northern Deanery*. Postgraduate Institute for Medicine and Dentistry, Newcastle upon Tyne.

11 Southgate L and Pringle M (1999) Revalidation in the United Kingdom: general principles based on experience in general practice. *BMJ*. **319**: 1180–3.

12 www.revalidationuk.info (accessed 5 November 2002).

13 www.doh.gov.uk/healthandsafety/gpguidance.htm (accessed 6 November 2002).

14 Sanderson P (2000) *Use of local medical committee counselling services in Northumberland* (personal communication).

15 Taylor GB and Sloan R (2003) Yorkshire: ready to meet the challenge of supervision in the twenty-first century? *Educ Prim Care.* **14**: 230–2.

16 Rotherham G, Martin D, Joesbury H *et al.* (1997) *Measures to Assess GPs Whose Performance Gives Cause for Concern.* University of Sheffield, Sheffield.

17 National Clinical Assessment Authority (2002) *Handbook for the Prototype Phase: general practice in England.* National Clinical Assessment Authority, London.

18 General Medical Council (1997) *The Performance Procedures: a guide to the new arrangements.* General Medical Council, London.

CHAPTER 15

Continuing professional development

Janet Grant

This chapter describes how continuing professional development (CPD) is central to clinical governance and needs to be managed. Effective CPD involves assessing educational needs, learning in a variety of different ways, and implementing and reinforcing that learning.

With the advent of clinical governance in primary care, continuing professional development (CPD) has moved centre-stage. As an important part of the risk management and quality assurance responsibilities of primary care trusts, practices and individual clinicians, the way in which CPD is managed in primary care is a subject of interest to users, providers and managers of primary healthcare services.

The new framework for CPD has been laid out clearly in *A First-Class Service*[1] and in the Chief Medical Officer's review of CPD in general practice.[2] The framework is consistent both with research on the effectiveness of CPD and with professional needs and approaches to continuing education.[3] It is generic, and it can and should be used to plan managed CPD for all members of the primary care team. The challenge set by the framework is not to develop new ways of learning in primary care, but rather to put into place a management process that will support the CPD that is undertaken and make it evident and relevant.

Continuing professional development, appraisal and revalidation

Continuing professional development, seen as a means of quality assuring patient care, has inevitably become intermixed with the revalidation of doctors. Likewise, the appraisals which were introduced as a means of helping individual clinicians to reflect on their own practice and to identify and act on their learning needs have also become part and parcel of revalidation. Thus revalidation, CPD and appraisal are now very much part of the same agenda, as shown in Figure 15.1.

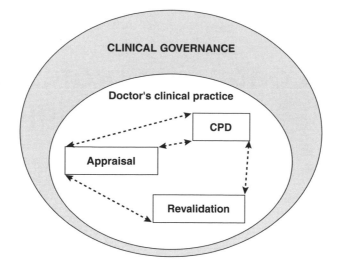

Figure 15.1 The link between clinical governance and appraisal, CPD and revalidation.

Appraisal

Formal appraisals appeared with the introduction across the NHS of clinical governance as outlined in the 1998 document *A First-Class Service: quality in the new NHS*.[1] This was reinforced in 1999 in the proposals for *Supporting Doctors, Protecting Patients*,[4] which addressed how to prevent, identify and deal with poor clinical performance. Appraisal therefore has both an educational role and a quality assurance role. These roles might or might not be seen as compatible.

Revalidation

As part of overall quality assurance, all doctors will be subject to revalidation procedures. The GMC states that:

> Revalidation of a doctor's licence every five years will signify that the GMC is satisfied that the doctor remains fit to practise medicine. It will also mean that the GMC will have seen appropriate evidence that the doctor is complying with the parts of *Good Medical Practice* relevant to his or her practice, as well as keeping up to date. For most doctors, the summary outputs from their annual appraisals will provide suitable and sufficient evidence for revalidation.

That evidence, and therefore appraisal, will be set against the seven headings set out in the GMC guidance *Good Medical Practice*.[5] GMC guidance for appraisal for revalidation is given as follows:

> During the appraisal, evidence being collected should help to identify any shortcomings in the doctor's performance, which can be addressed.

However, if there is serious concern that the doctor poses a risk to themselves or to patients, they should be referred to the GMC immediately.

It is clear then that appraisal, revalidation, clinical governance and CPD are all closely linked – and to make that linkage work smoothly for all purposes, a system for managing CPD must be found.

What is managed continuing professional development?

CPD vs. CME

Until recently, the learning that doctors undertook once they had completed their training was called continuing medical education (CME). However, three main factors have militated against the use of this term:

- the content areas that doctors now study
- the learning that clinicians share with other members of the healthcare team
- the need to make continuing education effective in developing and assuring standards of practice.

Although doctors will always continue to learn more about clinical medicine throughout their working lives, and to refine and develop their skills in this area, clinicians increasingly need to address areas that are not clinical at all. These might include information technology, management, audit and educational skills, and they are professional rather than purely medical matters.

Doctors increasingly share areas of their continuing professional development with other members of the healthcare team. National interest groups and societies (e.g. in asthma or diabetes) have a multiprofessional membership. In practices, questions of management and some aspects of practice policy will be shared by the team as a whole or by certain members of the team. As far as Government guidelines are concerned, the framework for CPD that is offered is one that can be applied to all members of the primary care team and to practices as a whole. It is therefore a framework that is designed for CPD, not for the continuing education of only one discipline. Systems of continuing education which simply ask for proof or an account of education undertaken do nothing to ensure that this education is either derived from or feeds back into practice. This means that neither the individual nor the health service can be confident that educational time has been well spent. If education is to be linked to CPD, then it must be approached, planned and managed more effectively. The emphasis will shift from isolated education to education as part of CPD.

CPD is accordingly defined in *A First-Class Service* as follows:

> a process of lifelong learning for all individuals and teams which meets the needs of patients and delivers the health outcomes and healthcare priorities of the NHS, and which enables professionals to expand and fulfil their potential.[1]

Managed CPD

Despite the existence of systems that have not required it, many doctors have assessed their own learning needs, undertaken learning relevant to those needs, and brought that learning back to the practice so that it influences the quality of patient care or organisation within the practice. However, it cannot be said that this has been the norm everywhere.

With clinical governance comes the need to ensure that all aspects of a clinician's work, and the work of the team, contribute towards a service of increasing quality, as the definition of clinical governance implies.[1]

The term 'accountable' in the definition makes it clear that if CPD is a significant part of clinical governance, then it is also a part that must be managed properly and openly, just as all other aspects of healthcare provision and organisation will be accountable and managed. In relation to that management, it is asserted that CPD programmes are best managed locally to meet both local service needs and those of individual professionals.[1]

Therefore:

> Health professionals, professional bodies and local employers need to discuss a locally based approach to CPD, centred on the service development needs of the local community and the learning needs of the individual.

Managed CPD and clinical governance

A First-Class Service stated that clinical governance provided the framework for a more coherent approach to local CPD, which would in turn support improvements in service quality.[1]

Its recommendations were quite explicit with regard to where CPD fitted into the clinical governance and quality framework. The importance of CPD and its role in quality assurance was reinforced by a recommendation that primary care groups should nominate a senior professional to take the lead on clinical standards and professional development, as part of the group's overall responsibility to demonstrate that quality of care is important.

The following specific points were made about CPD in relation to clinical governance.

- It must play a key part in improving quality.
- Individual health professionals and NHS employers should value CPD.
- CPD programmes should meet the learning needs of individual health professionals as well as the wider development needs of the service.
- Professional bodies should support effective CPD and promote lifelong learning.
- Much good CPD is already in practice throughout the NHS.
- CPD is essential to the development and support of clinical governance.
- CPD programmes are best managed locally to meet the needs of individuals and the service. This might include innovative approaches to work-based learning.
- The CPD cycle has five stages (*see* Box 15.1).
- Employers must recognise the value of appropriately managed CPD programmes in attracting, motivating and retaining high-calibre staff.

- Personal development plans (PDPs) should be developed by individuals in discussion with colleagues locally, perhaps in the context of performance appraisal.
- PDPs should take into account different preferred ways of learning, and should take full advantage of opportunities to learn on the job.
- Individual PDPs should be complemented by organisational development plans.
- The majority of health professionals should have PDPs in place by April 2000.

Box 15.1 Five stages of the CPD cycle

1 Assessment of individual and organisational needs
2 Making personal development plans (PDPs)
3 Implementation
4 Reinforcement and dissemination
5 Review of the effectiveness of the CPD intervention

What does managed CPD involve?

From the above, and from what is known about the effectiveness of CPD, we can state what managed CPD should mean in practice.

1 Each member of the primary care team should prepare a PDP.
2 This plan should record the following:
   - the need for the CPD to be undertaken
   - what the CPD will be
   - how that CPD will be reinforced and disseminated locally to show its effectiveness.
3 The PDP should take into account the needs of the individual and of the service.
4 The PDP should be prepared jointly by the individual and an appropriate colleague.
5 The PDP should form part of the practice professional development plan (PPDP), and so should be open to scrutiny and monitoring.

What makes continuing professional development effective?

Before describing the nature of managed CPD in primary care in more detail, it is important to appreciate that there is an evidential basis for it.

The literature review[3] undertaken for the Chief Medical Officer in preparation for the *Review of Continuing Professional Development in General Practice* reached the following conclusions.

1 The key to effectiveness of CPD is not to be found in the learning methods adopted.

2 There is not a best learning method, and there is no best approach to learning for CPD.
3 Instead, the key to effectiveness is to make sure that the process of CPD is managed effectively and has the following components:
   • *a stated reason* for the CPD to be undertaken. This might be specific (e.g. a need to develop a new skill) or it might be a general professional reason (e.g. a wish to undertake general professional updating with colleagues at a conference). It might also arise from the needs of the service (e.g. to develop the skill to offer new areas of care to patients)
   • *an identified method of learning*, which might be formal or informal
   • *some follow-up* after the CPD for reinforcement and dissemination of the learning, which can also demonstrate its benefits. This might include actions such as reporting back to colleagues, developing new services, demonstrating new skills or simply feeling more confident.

These conclusions match those of Davis *et al.*[6] in their review of randomised controlled trials of CPD interventions. Davis *et al.* elaborated on other reasons for success, and concluded that, in general, change was more likely to occur if:

• a needs assessment had been conducted
• the education was linked to practice
• the educational activity was undertaken as a result of personal incentive rather than some other influence
• there were reinforcing features after the educational event itself.

This is not to imply that all education should be based on identified specific needs. General professional continuing education, such as the large conference that covers many topics, is an important part of CPD. If all education was to be specific and based on rigid needs assessment, the profession would be narrow in its perspective and its development.

Implications

The implications of the review are as follows:

1 A managed process for CPD must be developed at the practice level.
2 The *process* of CPD should be monitored and rewarded, rather than the hours taken up by it.
3 The managed process must display the following characteristics of effectiveness:
   • a stated reason for undertaking the intended CPD (i.e. a statement of learning needs and interests)
   • an identified learning method (formal or informal)
   • a plan for reinforcing and disseminating the learning and demonstrating its effectiveness
   • a plan for review of the individual's PDP.

These implications are at the heart of the managed CPD that clinical governance requires.

Managed CPD in primary care

The principles of managed CPD apply to both primary and secondary care settings. In both cases, managed CPD must encompass the needs and interests of both the individual and the service. In hospitals, this can be achieved by integrating individual PDPs for CPD with the unit business plan. The equivalent of the unit business plan in primary care is sometimes called the *practice strategic plan*. However, in primary care where the educational needs of the whole team have been emphasised, a further planning stage is required to cover that whole team. This stage is summarised in the practice professional development plan (PPDP), as recommended in the Chief Medical Officer's report.[2] The levels of planning for CPD that are therefore recommended for primary care can be represented diagramatically as shown in Figure 15.2.

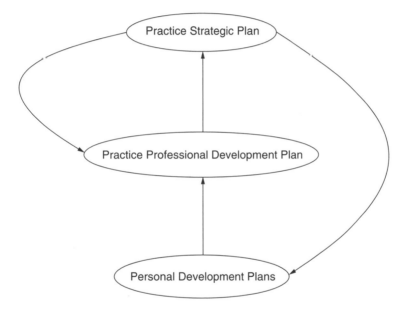

Figure 15.2   CPD planning in primary care.

The practice professional development plan (PPDP)

The PPDP addresses the learning needs of the whole practice and everyone in it. In essence it is the educational plan for the practice based on service development plans, local and national objectives and identified educational needs.

The PPDP is therefore practice based and should include an indication not only of what learning is required and planned for the practice, but also of how its effect would be demonstrated. Thus the PPDP is partially based on the practice strategic plan (or business plan), and feeds into that plan (*see* Box 15.2).

Box 15.2   Factors to be taken into account in PPDPs

- Service developments
- Clinical audit results
- Local and individual needs
- Local and national priorities
- User and carer involvement

The PPDP will allow practices to identify where both multiprofessional and uniprofessional learning is required.

The personal development plan (PDP)

In primary care, in common with all branches of the health service, the majority of staff were expected to have had a PDP by April 2000. The PDP must be a comprehensive document that records the outcome of appraisal, discussion of educational needs with a colleague or other forms of educational needs assessment. It must be sufficiently detailed to be a clear part of the PPDP and to be monitored for professional or employment reasons. It is the main professional record of the individual's activities in keeping up to date and ensuring the standard and quality of the service provided. The PDP is an instrumental part of clinical governance and professional maintenance of standards, and it is a key part of doctors' revalidation procedures.

A PDP should contain sections that record the following information:

- what the planned CPD activity is
- its intended date of completion
- how the educational need was identified
- the reinforcement and dissemination activities planned after the CPD itself is completed
- the dates of completion of the plans.

Fulfilment of the PDP can then be monitored.

An example of a PDP form is shown in Figure 15.3.

The stages of managed continuing professional development: identifying educational needs, learning and follow-up

There are three stages of managed CPD that the individual clinician will follow, namely needs identification, learning and follow-up (i.e. reinforcement, dissemination and demonstrating effectiveness).

The review of the effectiveness of CPD shows that these three stages are already being undertaken by many practitioners in many different ways, and that these

PERSONAL DEVELOPMENT PLAN

DOCTOR:

PRACTICE:

GMC NUMBER:

DATE:

PLAN FOR PERIOD: To

PROPOSALS DISCUSSED WITH: DATE OF DISCUSSION:

Description and intended date	Date completed	Signed by colleague [Date]
1. Proposed CPD activity Intended date:		Date:
How need was identified:		Date:
How CPD will be reinforced, and disseminated, showing effectiveness:		Date:
2. Proposed CPD activity Intended date:		Date:
How need was identified:		Date:
How CPD will be reinforced, and disseminated, showing effectiveness:		Date:

A copy of this form should be lodged in the Practice Strategic Plan and be retained for future use in relation to monitoring.

Figure 15.3   Personal development plan.

three stages together will ensure that CPD is effective both for individuals and for primary care teams. Preparation of the PDP will enable practitioners to demonstrate this fact and to consider new methods of effecting these stages.

A research and development project has identified and described the various ways in which doctors are already undertaking these three stages of managed CPD. The following examples are taken from the report of that project.[7]

Methods of needs assessment

A total of 48 methods of needs assessment have been identified, as shown in Table 15.1.

Table 15.1 Methods of needs assessment used in medicine

The clinician's own experiences in direct patient care
- Blind spots
- Clinically generated 'unknowns'
- Competence standards
- Diaries
- Difficulties arising in practice
- Innovations in practice
- Knowledgeable patients
- Mistakes
- Other disciplines
- Patients' complaints and feedback
- Post-mortems and the clinicopathological conference
- Patients' unmet needs (PUNs) and doctors' educational needs (DENs)
- Reflection on practical experience

Interactions within the clinical team and department
- Clinical meetings (departmental and grand rounds)
- Department business plan
- Department educational meetings
- External recruitment
- Junior staff
- Management roles
- Mentoring

Non-clinical activities
- Academic activities
- Conferences
- International visits
- Journal articles
- Medico-legal cases
- Press and media
- Professional conversations
- Research

continued

Table 15.1   Continued

- Teaching
- Patient satisfaction surveys
- Risk assessment

Formal approaches to quality management and risk assessment
- Audit
- Morbidity patterns
- Patient adverse events

Specific activities directed at needs assessment
- Critical incident analysis
- Gap analysis
- Objective tests of knowledge and skill
- Observation
- Revalidation systems
- Self-assessment
- Video assessment of performance

Peer review
- External
- Informal (of the individual doctor)
- Internal
- Multidisciplinary
- Physician assessment

The following unusual methods might require some description.

PUNs and DENs
This method has been developed and used in general practice.

- PUNs are patients' unmet needs.
- DENs are doctors' educational needs.

Richard Eve from Taunton, who developed this approach, recommends that a clinician collects PUNs during a set number of surgeries (outpatients, ward rounds, lists) simply by asking after each patient or session 'Was I equipped to meet the patient's needs? Could I have done better?'. Any clinician who thinks for a moment will be able to list many ways in which his or her practice has changed over the years. New drugs, new technology and equipment, and new methods, procedures and techniques are always being introduced. Along with these comes the need to learn to use them properly and well. Acquiring the training or education to do this should be a high priority and properly planned. A note should be made of the answers to these questions – these will be the PUNs. Thus an area or areas will be identified that might benefit from further learning or development – these will be the DENs. Eve points out that some PUNs will not be met by education, but by changes elsewhere (e.g. in organisation or administration). For CPD, it is necessary to identify those PUNs that truly indicate a DEN, and then to act on them.

Professional conversations

Clinicians spend their working life in a rich professional learning environment that is dominated by discussion of patients and of practice. Clinicians in all disciplines discuss their own patients with other clinicians, whose views they seek. They discuss shared patients as well as others' patients and experiences. These informal professional conversations are as much a part of learning and identifying learning needs as any other type of more formal approach to needs assessment. Such professional conversations contain feedback on performance in relation to specific patients when the management or outcome of treatment is discussed. They also contain new learning and open up new areas for learning, which are often followed up quite deliberately. Where this is the case, a learning need has been identified in a relevant and professional manner.

Gap analysis

This is based on the idea that 'a learning need is the gap between what you are now and what you want to be in regard to a particular set of competencies'.[8]

Gap analysis is undertaken by:

- defining the knowledge, skills, attitudes and competencies that are required to perform the relevant role to an excellent standard
- defining where you are in relation to each defined aspect. This can be done either by yourself or with the help of others.

Physician assessment

This is a particular variant of peer review which originated from the American Board of Internal Medicine[9] and was further developed by the Royal Australasian College of Physicians.[10] To undertake such an assessment, the doctor nominates a number of colleagues (say 15) to be assessors. Each is sent a standard rating form by the organising body (which could be the department, the trust or the Royal College) and asked to rate the doctor on various clinical skills and humanistic and other qualities. The ratings are fed back to the doctor, who takes educational action accordingly. The system shows encouraging levels of validity, reliability and acceptability, and has the advantage of credibility to the doctor who has nominated the assessors. This is a form of 360-degree appraisal.

Methods of learning

Research on the effectiveness of CPD shows that the method of learning which is adopted is not the crucial variable for effectiveness. Clinicians learn in a rich variety of ways, many of which are integrated into their daily professional activities. Learning in healthcare is often not a separate event from practice itself. Practitioners live in a rich learning environment where contact with other healthcare professionals, patients and other information sources is built into normal working. These are powerful sources of education and development both for the individual and for the team. *The Good CPD Guide*[7] describes over 40 such learning methods classified under the following headings:

- academic activities
- meetings
- learning from colleagues
- learning from practice
- technology-based learning and media
- management and quality-assurance processes
- specially arranged educational events.

The many methods identified under these headings will not be described further here. It is not the learning method itself that determines the effectiveness of the learning, but the stages of needs identification and reinforcement that precede and follow it. Nonetheless, it is important that every clinician is able to identify the various different ways of learning. They can then record them in their PDPs. In addition, the learning that occurs in such ways can perhaps be undertaken more deliberately, consciously and critically, and so more effectively.

Following up CPD: reinforcement, dissemination and demonstrating effectiveness

Following up CPD has three main purposes.

1 It reinforces the learning in the practice context.
2 It allows for dissemination of the learning to others in the practice.
3 It allows the overall effectiveness of the CPD to be assessed.

These three purposes differ in their intent. Reinforcement will ensure that the primary learning is strengthened by its rehearsal or revisiting in some way. Dissemination allows the learning to be shared with others, discussed and analysed. Both reinforcement and dissemination might involve application of the learning to change or develop practice. Demonstration of the overall effectiveness of the learning will often be a consequence or antecedent of the reinforcement and dissemination activities, but it might also be a special event.

Although the effectiveness of CPD can be demonstrated in many different ways, hardly any of these will be able to produce a measurable outcome, or a causal relationship between the education and the effect studied. This is so for a number of reasons.

- On some occasions the CPD will simply show that the clinician's practice is acceptable and does not need to be changed. The only 'measurable' outcome therefore might be increased confidence on the part of the clinician.
- Many important outcomes of education are unpredictable or, if they are predictable, are often unmeasurable (e.g. 'better team spirit').
- Education is often not an isolated event but occurs in parallel with other educational influences. Thus it is difficult to isolate the effects of that event.

- Where education is a discrete event, there are often many interfering variables between event and patient outcome that might either militate against or facilitate the observed outcome. Attribution of that outcome to the education will therefore be impossible. The problem of measuring outcomes has been discussed further by Grant and Stanton.[3]

Despite these difficulties, it should be remembered that the clinician's professional judgement of unmeasurable qualities can be as valuable and valid as quantitative data that can only measure the measurable, and thus often miss the important.

The Good CPD Guide discusses 41 different ways of following up learning (*see* Table 15.2). It is crucial that this stage of the managed CPD process is not omitted.

Table 15.2   Methods of following up CPD

1 Accreditation/certification of the individual	22 Networking
2 Accreditation of services	23 New services
3 Appraisal	24 Obsolete and inappropriate practice
4 Assessment of learning	25 Peer review of the doctor's CPD
5 Assessment results of trainees	26 Peer review of the medical team
6 Audit	27 Personal invigoration
7 Changes in person specification	28 Protection from successful litigation
8 Changing practice	29 Recruitment of medical staff
9 Clinical effectiveness	30 Reduction in burnout and early retirement
10 CPD credit points	31 Referrals to the doctor
11 Collaborative assessment	32 Remunerative benefit (discretionary points, merit awards, etc.)
12 Confidence levels	
13 Corporate image	33 Reporting back to colleagues
14 Decreasing professional isolation	34 Reputation as trainer
15 'Don't know' factor	35 Research
16 Educational culture	36 Risk management
17 Educational record and logbooks	37 Self-assessment
18 Effects on the team	38 Time-efficient working
19 Enhancing practice	39 Video assessment
20 Learning diaries	40 Video-stimulated recall
21 Learning portfolios	41 Written reports

Moving on

The advent of clinical governance affects every aspect of the management and delivery of healthcare. It demands changes in infrastructure and process. With regard to CPD, the role of GP tutors, for example, and the relationship between primary care trusts and the Directors of Postgraduate General Practice Education will require consideration. There are many strands to be interwoven and roles to be co-ordinated. Some of these can be resolved at a regional or local level, but other issues can only be resolved at a national level – primary among these is the new GP contract.

Discussions of this will need to address organisation and management issues, and funding streams and processes. A change of focus is required so that the successful implementation of well-managed CPD, with all of the features described here, is recognised by the funding arrangements. A funding system which implies that simple attendance at an educational event is good enough, regardless of need, quality or benefit to practitioner or practice, is no longer professionally acceptable. Of course, such events will still feature in the educational activities of GPs – there is nothing in managed CPD that precludes the doctor from learning in any particular way – but the educational event itself will no longer be the sole feature of education. Instead, that event will become part of a process of learning that starts with practice and returns to practice. It is this process, which is fundamental to clinical governance, that funding arrangements must now recognise.

Practical points

Note: The term CPD is preferred to CME, as it encompasses a broader content of learning and covers all professional groups.

- CPD is central to the implementation of clinical governance.
- CPD should be managed locally – at the primary care team level.
- PPDPs should incorporate PDPs for the whole team.
- The method that is used to learn is not as important as the process of assessing educational needs beforehand, and reinforcing and disseminating the learning afterwards.
- For CPD to be effective, it is vital to get the process right.

References

1   Department of Health (1998) *A First-Class Service: quality in the new NHS*. Department of Health, London.
2   Department of Health (1998) *A Review of Continuing Professional Development in General Practice: a report by the Chief Medical Officer*. Department of Health, London.
3   Grant J and Stanton F (1998) *The Effectiveness of Continuing Professional Development: a report for the Chief Medical Officer's Review of Continuing Professional Development in General Practice* (2e). Joint Centre for Education in Medicine, London.
4   Department of Health (1999) *Supporting Doctors, Protecting Patients*. Department of Health, London.
5   General Medical Council (2001) *Good Medical Practice* (3e). General Medical Council, London.
6   Davis DA, Thomson MA, Oxman AD and Haynes B (1995) Changing physician performance: a systematic review of the effect of continuing medical education strategies. *JAMA*. **247**: 700–5.
7   Grant J, Chambers E and Jackson G (1999) *The Good CPD Guide*. Reed Healthcare Publishing, Sutton.

8 Knowles N (1990) *The Adult Learner: a neglected species* (4e). Gulf Publishing Co., Houston, TX.

9 Ramsey PG, Carline JD, Inui TS, Larson EB, LoGerfo JP and Weinrich MD (1989) Predictive validity of certification by the American Board of Internal Medicine. *Ann Intern Med.* **110**: 719–26.

10 Paget NS, Newble DI, Saunders NS and Du J (1996) Physician assessment pilot study for the Royal Australasian College of Physicians. *J Contin Educ Health Prof.* **16**: 103–11.

CHAPTER 16

Developing leaders

Jamie Harrison

Leadership remains the most studied and least understood topic in all the social sciences.

Warren Bennis

This chapter explores how to develop leaders and leadership in primary care. In a time of change, the complementary roles of leadership and management are highlighted, and a pattern of servant leadership is suggested for the future.

Introduction

Primary care has not always been good at developing leaders. Certainly within traditional general practice the rule was that GPs led the organisation, with the doctor with the greatest seniority controlling the GPs – whether or not that individual was a skilled leader.

Thus team leadership was based purely on length of clinical experience (or time served in the practice), rather than on ability to lead. More recently, this hierarchical approach has been challenged by the introduction of executive partners and professionally trained practice managers into local practices, and by health authority managers working alongside GPs within commissioning groups and primary care trusts. Nevertheless, many GPs are cautious about being directed in how to do their work. Equally, they remain suspicious of those who seek to lead them. This partly reflects the fact that, historically, GPs have valued their independence, individualism and relative lack of accountability. As a result, they have found it difficult to reach a consensus in formulating policy matters, not least in how to respond to the Government's proposed contractual changes, notably in 1990.

This inability to find a common mind on matters of policy in tandem with an unwillingness to carry out concerted action suggests that, were they proverbial horses, GPs would never allow themselves to be led to water, and would certainly not agree to drink. Others in primary care may not be so fiercely individualistic, but they can be hampered by training and employment cultures that suppress initiative and independent thinking. Again this situation is changing, as nurses, managers and professionals allied to medicine are allowed to develop as independent practitioners, as well as leaders of uniprofessional teams.

The role of clinical governance in this area is complex. While seeking to balance a proper desire for greater professional freedom, there is a need for corporate accountability within multiprofessional primary care teams. And the world of primary care itself is changing rapidly. Teams will need good leadership if they are to cope with the rate of change, which – if anything – is accelerating.

What is leadership?

The new quality agenda[1] puts added pressure on primary care teams who have, for whatever reason, failed to move with the times. Yet all practices and practitioners can do better. Clinical governance is suggested as the means by which everyone in primary care will improve. However, within the clinical governance agenda it is worth asking what will drive the various components described. Is effective leadership the necessary first mechanism, which will initially trigger and then guide and encourage the full set of governance mechanisms? Indeed, without leadership, will clinical governance get off the ground at all?

Professor John Kotter, from the Harvard Business School, reminds us that leadership is vital during times of change, and that it is different from management:

> Management is about coping with complexity. ... Leadership, by contrast, is about coping with change. ... More change demands more leadership.[2]

Thus primary care must come to accept that, in a rapidly changing environment, effective leadership will be increasingly necessary, and that better management on its own is insufficient to deal with the new quality agenda. For leadership is the means by which the quality agenda can be driven forward, leaving it to management to solve the problems left in its wake (*see* Box 16.1). And we must never lose sight of the fact that 'leadership complements management; it doesn't replace it'.[2]

For Kotter, effective leaders should have the following attributes:

- vision, with the ability to formulate strategies
- ready access to a reservoir of support mechanisms with which to respond to changing situations for themselves and others
- the ability or charisma to increase motivation and build a team or teams.

How is leadership to be developed? And what makes a good leader?

Box 16.1   Differences between leadership and management

Leadership
- Develops strategy
- Copes with change
- Creates the team
- Increases motivation and inspires

Management
- Puts strategy into practice
- Copes with complexity
- Maintains the team
- Monitors and solves problems

How to develop as a leader

Ken Jarrold is clear that we learn about leadership from the example of others – through reading literature, hearing stories, seeing events in the news, and reflecting on our own experience of leadership and leaders within the NHS. For Jarrold, leadership is about service:

> If leadership is about showing the way, about knowing what to do next, about the courage to stand against, about giving people space, how do you do it? You lead by serving.[3]

He goes on to suggest five steps to those who are willing to grow as servant leaders.

- *Learn to listen* – to questions and requests for advice, for information, experience, wisdom and knowledge.
- *Keep thinking* – sort information; analyse and grapple with issues.
- *Foster sound judgement* – evaluate the situation and decide what is right.
- *Be clear* – explain your analysis and decision; people and organisations require clarity.
- *Be courageous* – this is not to be confused with arrogance; servant leaders need humility, but they also need courage – 'the power to stand against' (Peter Ackroyd).

For Jarrold, the last word in this area goes to David Wilkinson and Elaine Applebee, for whom the emphasis is on the need for courage in leadership, rather than simply charisma:

> Leaders communicate more by what they do, champion and support than by what they say. They are able to substantially increase the stock of leadership across the system, generating a wide commitment to act, learn and take risks. It is feedback from this that in turn sustains effective leaders. It is important that leaders find their own styles, and can act with a range of styles contingent upon the situation. Above all, they need to be able to live and work with paradox, dilemmas and uncertainty – both their own and others.[4]

Yet leaders must find ways in which to engage with those whom they are called upon to lead. The type of leadership style that they adopt will profoundly influence their relationship with a team or organisation, and thus play a major role in the effectiveness of the whole enterprise.

Leadership style

Leadership style can range from authoritarian to democratic, to *laissez-faire*. In the authoritarian style, the leader makes the decisions. In the democratic style, the group decides by majority vote. In the *laissez-faire* approach, the leader allows individuals to decide for themselves, or not to decide at all – depending on how the team or organisation feels at the time.[5]

How leaders lead depends on the context, the occasion and their personal beliefs about leadership. The most dominant of these is the leader's own personal value system. Leaders who value status and position will resent any attempts to undermine their authority and power. Leaders who see themselves as servants will not.

Equally, within teams there will be expectations of how the leader should lead. If a team expects firm leadership, its members may block the leader's attempts to encourage participation in decision making – after all, that is the leader's job. Young teams, and newly formulated organisations such as primary care group boards and clinical governance subgroups, may find their members drawn from a wide range of professional and other backgrounds. Care will be needed initially to give such groupings direction. In a new situation, it is unwise to try to use highly participative approaches too soon.

It is also important to tailor leadership style to the context. However democratic the clinical team, during a cardiac arrest it is inappropriate to take a vote on the dose of adrenaline to be administered. Someone needs to take charge and give the orders. Once the emergency is over, there will be time to reflect together on the next course of action.

The more mature the team and its leader, the more flexible and innovative the leadership can be, moving easily between directive, democratic and easygoing styles as and when the situation demands. Figure 16.1 illustrates the various hierarchies of leadership that are observed in practice within organisations, with the relative degree of power exercised by the leader and by team members shown on the right-hand side of the figure.

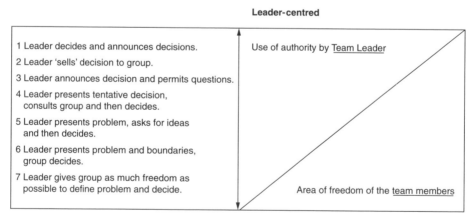

Leader-centred

1 Leader decides and announces decisions.

2 Leader 'sells' decision to group.

3 Leader announces decision and permits questions.

4 Leader presents tentative decision, consults group and then decides.

5 Leader presents problem, asks for ideas and then decides.

6 Leader presents problem and boundaries, group decides.

7 Leader gives group as much freedom as possible to define problem and decide.

Use of authority by Team Leader

Area of freedom of the team members

Team-centred

Figure 16.1 Leadership styles (based on the Tannenbaum Schmidt model[5]).

David Cormack concludes that there are five general principles with regard to leadership style.

- There is probably no single right style of leader behaviour.
- Effective leaders base their behaviour on the context in which they find themselves.

- Effective leaders can modify their leadership style to fit the demands of the situation.
- Team members become confused and frustrated when leaders behave differently to how they expect their leader to lead.
- Effective leaders of mature teams operate as near to the group-centred end of the continuum of power sharing as is possible in any one situation.

Leaders may find it helpful to reflect on their own preferred leadership style. Whatever that may be, the goal of leadership remains the same – to achieve results, to achieve success in the team's or organisation's chosen field. For primary care, this means meeting the needs of patients in an accessible, comprehensive, co-ordinated and continuing way.

Leadership in primary care

Leaders in primary care work at the sharp end of the health service, being required not only to manage change, but also to lead it. This requires the ability to shape, share and articulate vision and strategy, as well as excellent communication skills, drive and enthusiasm, political awareness and the ability to motivate and support others. As Tim van Zwanenberg has put it, such leaders:

> must rise above parochial and professional vested interests. Leadership is neither wholly an innate quality nor wholly a learned skill. Some have an aptitude to become leaders, and they need opportunities to develop the appropriate skills.[6]

The challenge to primary care is how to identify, train and nurture such leaders. Primary care trust clinical governance leads have already articulated their desire for support in this area (*see* Box 16.2).

Clinical governance leads in primary care groups obviously feel the need to develop skills in both management and leadership, notably in strategic thinking,

---

Box 16.2 Development needs identified by primary care group clinical governance leads[7]

- Strategic thinking
- Motivation
- Team leadership   *Leadership skills*
- Change management

- Negotiation
- The development of systems for measuring care
- Dissemination
- Marketing   *Management skills*
- Risk management

motivation, team leadership and change management. Interviews with GPs yielded similar results, with a comment that 'there was nothing in general practitioner training about team development or leadership, and that this was a considerable omission in their development which needed to be addressed'.[7]

Strategic thinking

Since the function of leadership is to produce change, setting the direction of that change is fundamental. Setting direction is not the same as planning, or even long-term planning, although the two are often confused. Rather, planning is a management process that is deductive in nature and designed to produce orderly results, not change.

> Setting a direction is more inductive. Leaders gather a broad range of data and look for patterns, relationships and linkages that help explain things. What's more, the direction-setting aspect of leadership does not produce plans; it creates vision and strategies.[2]

Kotter goes on to discuss the idea of how to develop a strategy:

> Nor do visions and strategies have to be brilliantly innovative; in fact, some of the best are not. Effective (business) visions regularly have an almost mundane quality, usually consisting of ideas that are already well known. The particular combination of the ideas may be new, but sometimes even that is not the case.

In the context of primary care, there are plenty of good ideas, innovations and practical strategies already in use somewhere in the UK. There is no need to reinvent the wheel. What is crucial is to become aware of this rich seam of options, and to harness the most useful and appropriate ones to inform local strategies. This process must also take into account the needs of the stakeholders (health authorities, primary care staff and patients).

Charles Handy describes the characteristics necessary for a strategy or vision to be effective, making the point that 'a leader shapes and shares a vision which gives point to the work of others'[8] (*see* Box 16.3).

Box 16.3 Characteristics of an effective vision or strategy

- It must be different.
- It must make sense to others.
- It must stretch people's imagination but also be achievable.
- It must be understandable.
- It must be lived by the leader.
- It must be believed in and enacted by the whole team.

After Handy[8]

Motivation

Motivation comes from within, from the feelings and attitudes that are experienced in response to basic needs. Whatever the popular view, you cannot in fact 'motivate' someone else. However, you can create situations in which they or others will be motivated.

The work of Abraham Maslow[9] describes five basic human needs – to have, to be, to do, to love and to grow. His analysis contains the notion of a hierarchy of needs, in that individuals vary both in their perceived 'basic' needs and in what motivates them beyond their minimum requirements for survival.

The leader's role is to provide an environment in which people are motivated – where team members are able to satisfy their needs while also doing what the team requires of them. A model of motivation is illustrated in Figure 16.2.

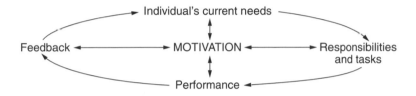

Figure 16.2 A model of motivation.

Some people are motivated by attractive working conditions, extra holidays and financial rewards, while others are motivated by the knowledge that they are doing a good job, have status in the team and are valued. The art of the team leader in primary care is to identify what motivates each individual team member, creating the right atmosphere, opportunities and incentives for that person to develop.

Team leadership

Team leadership is closely allied to creating a work environment that helps individuals to be motivated and to perform well. Any one individual's current needs will change from time to time as their domestic circumstances and work contexts change. New team members will first need to gain acceptance within the team. As they become established, they will need new challenges and greater responsibility. Leaders need to facilitate this.

The role and effectiveness of each team member will need regular clarification if stagnation and confusion are to be avoided. The team leader has the responsibility to ensure that all team members are clear about their respective roles within the organisation, how they fit in with colleagues, what the overall strategy is and how they are performing (both individually and as a unit). This involves leaders setting targets and giving team members properly resourced opportunities to perform, with good feedback and formal appraisal.

It goes without saying that good communication is essential if effective leadership is to thrive. Leaders in primary care need to trust their team members, act with integrity, tell the truth, welcome constructive comment and criticism, and lead by example. Such leaders will need to be directive on occasions, take responsibility, and make difficult decisions when necessary.

Change management

Change is a natural process, although recently the health service seems to have had more than its fair share. For many in primary care, change is difficult. As we have already noted, leadership is about coping with change, so it must therefore be about helping to manage the changes that are thrust upon colleagues and team members.

Change occurs for a number of reasons. In primary care, change can result from any of the following:

- national initiatives and the imposition of new NHS frameworks (e.g. clinical governance)
- the formation of new local organisational structures (e.g. primary care groups)
- changes to primary care team personnel (e.g. one health visitor leaves and is replaced by another)
- changes to the team's character (e.g. the team grows tired and stale)
- new demands on the team's services (e.g. added work from early hospital discharges).

All of these changes must be managed – that is, they must be handled in a way that moves the team forward in pursuit of its aims. In order to achieve this, leaders must continue to review strategy, resource allocation, methods of monitoring and workload. Promoting communication, team-member training, learning from experience and learning from others in a similar situation would also seem to be essential.

Leadership in primary care trusts and primary care teams

Primary care trusts

Primary care trusts depend on board chairs, chief executives and clinical governance leads. Their capacity to develop as leaders depends on their innate ability, a commitment to the leadership task, appropriate training, the support and encouragement of colleagues, and the provision of adequate time, personnel and financial resources.

The roles of chair and chief executive are obviously different, although both require leadership skills. The primary care trust itself is a federation of organisations, and as such demands a different type of leadership to a single organisational structure. Negotiation will be important, as well as clarity of strategic thinking and effective communication.

The framework for the first years of clinical governance includes establishing leadership in primary care trusts.[10] The essential issues for leaders are those of inclusivity, openness, clarity, co-operation, commitment, communication and accountability. Lay board members have a key role to play in reviewing the effectiveness of such leadership, and in acting as a bridge for leaders to the wider community.

Primary care trust clinical governance leads will need both to build a team within their governance subgroups and to draw together the governance leads within the individual primary care teams. This will require skill in diplomacy, a clear strategy and the ability to listen. Being realistic about what is achievable, allied to creating an environment that motivates others, would also appear to be necessary.

In subsequent years, primary care trusts will need to develop leadership that learns from its own experiences, reflects on the wisdom of others, identifies new leaders locally, thinks strategically (especially about primary care trust formation), and builds up and develops the infrastructure of primary care. It might be worth remembering Tim van Zwanenberg's key strategic themes for tomorrow's GP – these themes have validity for all in primary care (*see* Box 16.4).

Box 16.4   Strategic themes for primary care[6]

Leadership
- Vision
- Communication skills
- Motivating others
- Above vested interests

Scholarship
- Learning valued
- Research and teaching
- Higher qualifications

Fellowship
- Mutual support
- Flexible careers
- Mentoring

Primary care teams

Leadership within primary care teams will continue to be carried out predominantly by doctors. This reflects a combination of their status, ownership of practice premises and the fact that many primary care staff are currently employees of GP partnerships.

However, the situation is changing. Nurse leadership within Personal Medical Services (PMS) schemes and the appointment of nurses as primary care group clinical governance leads points one way for the future. There is no reason why practice nurses, district nurses or health visitors should not be primary care team governance leads. Indeed, this is already happening.

Yet most clearly a culture of leadership needs to be created within practices and primary care teams. Sadly, the on-the-job experiences of many people actually seem to undermine their development as leaders. Recruiting those with leadership potential is one step in the right direction.

Another is to manage the career and work patterns of established team members by creating challenging opportunities, allowing exposure to a wide range of leaders and contexts, and broadening experience both within and beyond the health service (through sabbaticals both at home and abroad, secondment to non-NHS organisations and involvement in networking ventures such as Common Purpose).

These wide experiences teach people about life, how others lead, how society operates and how patients think in the world outside the NHS. More importantly, they also teach people in primary care teams something about both the difficulty of leadership and its potential for producing change.

Encouraging tomorrow's leaders in primary care

Leadership in primary care is at a crossroads. As more is asked of primary care by the Government, patients, managers and clinical staff, exciting new possibilities present themselves. As Ken Jarrold comments:

> We need to recognise and encourage the leaders in primary care. The most able leaders in primary care sustain both local communities and the NHS. The most successful leaders of primary care groups will have a strong claim to leadership in the NHS.[3]

Can primary care rise to the challenge? Will the leaders of primary care – to be found within primary care groups, primary care teams, uniprofessional local organisations (local medical committees, the Royal College of Nursing, the Royal College of General Practitioners and their equivalents), undergraduate and postgraduate university departments, and health authority primary care directorates – grasp the opportunities that are offered by the new quality agenda? If so, they must recognise that there are other leaders within the NHS who demand their respect, with whom they can work and from whom they can learn (*see* Box 16.5).

Box 16.5   Other leaders in the NHS

- Patient and carer leaders
- Public leaders (local communities)
- Political leaders
- NHS trade-union leaders
- NHS management leaders
- Secondary-care leaders

After Jarrold[3]

Identifying and training tomorrow's leaders is an ongoing task which will need imagination, resources (from both inside and outside the NHS) and time. Moreover, such leaders must not lose sight of the primary purpose of primary care, which is to respond appropriately to the needs of patients and their carers. For those working in primary care in the NHS (an organisation funded by taxation, with its ethos firmly that of public service), it may be wise to remember how health service leaders differ from senior managers in strictly commercial ventures, such as a public limited company (plc), and to respond accordingly (*see* Box 16.6).

Box 16.6   Differences between public and private sector leaders

NHS leaders
- Value diversity of style across teams
- Non-profit ethos
- Respect and care for all equally
- Decentralise power (subsidiarity)
- *End* – healthy people

Managing directors (plc)
- Impose corporate culture
- Profit maximisation
- Target specific consumer groups
- Centralise decision making
- *End* – healthy profit

Developing leaders in primary care will continue to be both demanding and rewarding. To be truly effective, leaders will need to receive the title 'leader' from their organisation and also to earn the right to lead, by their example. No leader will gain the following of a team without first showing and experiencing a personal commitment to the team itself, its individual members and the task that is set before it, all lived out in the spirit of service:

> The leader must know that he is most deeply committed to his followers, most heavily laden with responsibility towards the orders of life, in fact quite simply a servant.[11]

Ultimately, primary care must create leaders and leadership if it is to develop and change the way in which its teams and organisations function, thereby bringing benefit to all – patients, clinicians and managers alike. Where a corporate culture exists that values effective servant leadership and strives to maintain and further such leadership, the organisation concerned will truly flourish.

Developing such a culture is the work of a leader. Within the complexity of contemporary primary care, that would seem to be an essential task. Indeed, institutionalising a leadership-centred culture could be seen as the ultimate act of leadership.

Practical points

- Leadership is about creating and coping with change.
- Management is about coping with complexity.
- Leadership is required to get clinical governance off the ground, whereas management is required to implement its many components.
- Leaders adopt different styles – the best leaders use the style appropriate for the situation.
- In primary care, the style of servant-leader may allow both the formulation of strategy and the creation of an environment in which team members are motivated.
- There is a need to identify and nurture primary care leaders of the future.

References

1   Department of Health (1998) *A First-Class Service: quality in the new NHS*. Department of Health, London.
2   Kotter JP (1999) *What Leaders Really Do.* Harvard Business Review Books, Cambridge, MA.
3   Jarrold K (1998) Servants and leaders: leadership in the NHS. In: *York Symposium on Health: a report of the fourth symposium held at the University of York, 30 July 1998.* Department of Health Studies, University of York.
4   Wilkinson D and Applebee E (1999) *Implementing Holistic Government: joined-up action on the ground.* Policy Press, University of Bristol, Bristol.
5   Cormack D (1987) *Team Spirit: people working with people.* MARC Europe, Bromley. (For a more detailed analysis of leadership styles, the reader should consult Schein EH (1988) *Organizational Psychology.* Prentice-Hall, Englewood Cliffs, NJ.)
6   van Zwanenberg T (2002) GP tomorrow. In: J Harrison and T van Zwanenberg (eds) *GP Tomorrow.* Radcliffe Medical Press, Oxford.
7   Firth-Cozens J (1999) *Report on Clinical Governance Development Needs in Health Service Staff.* University of Northumbria, Newcastle upon Tyne.
8   Handy C (1991) *The Age of Unreason.* Arrow Business Books, London.
9   Maslow A (1954) *Motivation and Personality.* Harper and Row, New York.
10 Department of Health (1999) *Clinical Governance: quality in the new NHS*. Department of Health, London.
11 Bonhoeffer D (1965) *No Rusty Swords: letters, lectures and notes 1928–1936.* Collins, London.

CHAPTER 17

Developing teamwork

Pauline Pearson

This chapter describes how good teamwork, particularly within the primary healthcare team, contributes to the success of patient care.

Primary healthcare teams: past, present and future

The broad idea of the primary healthcare team has been well established for decades, particularly since the 1980s, when the Harding Report[1] examined how healthcare was delivered in a community setting and suggested how it might relate to better outcomes for patients. However, the specific components need to be teased out here. The primary healthcare team is often referred to as the primary care team, or even as the general practice team (the latter term was more common two or more decades ago), but muddled and inexact terminology reflects a general sloppiness of thought about what might be meant by the phrase. One way of clarifying what we are talking about might be to look at the specific words that are being used here.

- *Primary* – in the World Health Organization (WHO) Alma Ata statement,[2] *primary* healthcare is so called because it is the *first* point of access to healthcare for the majority of the population. Although this concept has broadened to incorporate *NHS Direct* and Walk-In Centres, as well as to acknowledge the importance of a variety of ambulatory care facilities, general-practice-based care remains the first point of access to healthcare for the vast majority of people in the UK.
- *Health* – this is defined in the same WHO statement as 'a state of complete physical, social and psychological well-being' (a state that is rarely attained). It is more commonly understood by lay people as not being ill, and functioning effectively and being happy. It is doubtful how closely the day-to-day aspirations of community health professionals relate to the achievement of this concept.
- *Care* – this is another slippery concept which has been discussed by many authors,[3-5] but which suggests an active engagement. The *Oxford English Dictionary* suggests that it means 'serious attention and thought'. As a verb, it means 'feel concern', or it may be used to mean 'attend to the well-being of' individuals or communities.
- *Team* – the final component is often seen in terms of a sporting or competitive team – that is, a group that is selected to work together to achieve a sporting or

other publicly recognised goal. In this context, where we are looking at a group of people, selected perhaps as individuals rather than for their contribution to the group working together, West and Poulton[6] talk about 'work groups'. For many people, the idea of a team involves a group of individuals inhabiting a single pitch or one health centre. A primary healthcare *team* might thus be a group that works together in some sense and has a clear identity – the X practice or the Y health centre – and a set of functions that are derived from and contribute to the achievement of clear organisational objectives related to the achievement of primary healthcare.

As we move forward in a context of significant change in NHS policy, we need to acknowledge the policy climate in which primary healthcare teams are functioning and in which they will continue to work. Particularly important is the modernisation of the NHS. The Government wants to convince people that it is listening to their concerns about the NHS and can get results – hence (I believe) the modernising agenda, travelling in the wake of an earlier tranche of change and focusing in particular on issues of pay and human resources. Where the workforce of primary and community care in particular is ageing fast, with large numbers of doctors, nurses and other healthcare workers due to retire in the next decade or so and recruitment not expanding fast enough to replace them, new models of practice and potentially new or reskilled team members will need to be developed. In addition, the Government is seeking to 'shift the balance of power',[7] make local clinicians more directly accountable to local people, and create (it hopes) seamless services that respond quickly to local need. Alongside this is a concern to ensure high quality and systematic standards of transparent and responsive governance. As well as the *Shifting the Balance of Power* programme, there has been substantial work on the importance of including patients within healthcare teams as participants, and in particular in the role of expert patients, as well as policy with regard to tackling health inequalities. Policy shifts then suggest that teams in the future may be rather different to those in the past, incorporating greater specialisation and delegation, new roles and more patient involvement.

Although many people will continue to work in patterns that have been broadly established for at least 5–10 years, and in many cases for longer, even here it is likely that the emphasis of their work will have changed during that time, and will continue to do so subtly and incrementally. At the same time, there will continue to be a mushrooming of 'new developments', rapidly becoming ubiquitous and thus in a way less 'new'. Examples of this type of mechanism could include people from a range of backgrounds working in Personal Medical Services (PMS) pilots with homeless people, people moving into Sure Start projects, those practising as nurse practitioners, GPs developing new roles in occupational health and public health or within primary care trusts, and a variety of therapists developing community outreach roles and direct-access clinics. Each of these represents a cluster of individuals trying out a particular way of working to deliver improved healthcare for local communities. Primary healthcare teams, whether traditional or new, will therefore need to ensure that they are capable not only of working together effectively, but also of responding flexibly to change.

Advantages of teamwork

Why organise work in groups? The reason is that throughout history human beings have found that there are advantages to collaboration and teamwork, whether as hunter-gatherers in the Stone Age or as health professionals in the twenty-first century. In the twentieth century much of the evidence for team functioning was examined by occupational psychologists and formalised. This evidence has been summarised by a number of writers in relation to team function, most notably by Michael West and his colleagues (*see*, for example, West and Poulton[6]), but will be briefly considered here.

One individual hunter alone would be unlikely to amass a 'bag' equivalent to the achievement of a group. This in itself is obvious. However, an effect similar to the well-known 'Hawthorn effect' (from organisational research), where the act of simply being observed improves performance, can also be identified. The awareness of being part of a team, and therefore competing within that team, appears to have led to the development of a conviction that the combination of individuals' performances will be exceeded by the group performance – that is, participants will each do better as part of a group.

Research has also suggested that groups make decisions better than individual members, at least as far as the average quality of decisions made by individual members (rated by experts external to the group) is concerned. This is perhaps unsurprising, given the greater pool of experience that can be drawn upon by the individuals concerned. In terms of holding on to that experience in a changing NHS, another advantage of teams, which is supported by evidence from research, is the capacity of such an organisation to maintain memories of what has been tried, and what has or has not worked. Where individuals forget or move on, a collective is able to recall experience, at least in a fragmentary way, over a longer period. There is evidence that primary healthcare teams based around general practice have expanded considerably in recent decades,[8] as in society in general groups have become larger and more complex (*see*, for example, the mean number of researchers listed in individual published papers in any medical journal in 1990 compared with 2000). As organisations have become larger and structurally more complex, people have recognised the need to work together in groups of manageable size, where objectives are co-ordinated and achievable. The achievement of organisational goals is also believed to be enhanced by such an approach.

What can go wrong?

Very often, despite the rhetoric, teams and groups fail to deliver improved outcomes over those that might be achieved by adding individual members together – indeed, sometimes they do worse! Psychologists have explored the reasons for this extensively, and have highlighted a number of possibilities. Although groups make better decisions than individual members, this only appears to be true as far as the average quality of decisions made by individual members is concerned. In any given group, there may be dominant and less creative individuals who are able by sheer force of personality to overwhelm lower-status, better-quality thinkers, or perhaps individuals whose contributions are lost or muffled due to lack of communication skills, or undue attention to conformity, or perhaps to gender effects.

Given the nature of most primary healthcare teams in which large numbers of relatively low-status women are (still) often working with a smaller number of high-status, confident and well-educated men, this is an area that requires active attention. Research suggests that even at their best, groups will often fail to achieve collective decisions of the quality that could be achieved by their most capable individual members.

Where there is a degree of cohesion within a group, a number of other psychological mechanisms can take hold. One which appears relatively predictable to the lay person is the tendency for members to move towards decisions that are relatively 'easy' in that they are immediately acceptable to the group, rather than to work towards what may be more difficult to achieve but may for various reasons be a better decision. In order to avoid this problem, the team will need a clear vision of where it is going and effective leadership. Another problem that may arise, particularly if the members of a group feel secure with one another, is for individuals to be willing to take greater risks as a collective, and thus to make more extreme decisions than would be the average of their members' decisions. Care in assessing and discussing risk is essential in order to combat this problem. Some research has also suggested that individuals may put less effort into their work if they believe that their efforts are combined with and masked by those of colleagues. This may sound very familiar to those who have worked in unevenly balanced teams, particularly in larger groups where lack of individual effort can often be hidden. Such problems will only be highlighted where close attention is paid to reviewing individual performance.

Developing and growing a team

Most often in the recent past, primary healthcare teams have grown gradually, changing their membership over a long period of time. However, with the current fast pace of change, increasing numbers of new and reformulated teams are likely to be formed, in PMS pilots on under-doctored estates, in community-based outreach teams, in Sure Start projects, and in the development of radically new roles within old teams. The teams themselves then need to be nurtured, and the environment and leadership within them must be facilitative, because practitioners cannot achieve success alone. Resourcing also needs to be adequate.

Probably the most crucial elements for developing a team will be first to develop a team identity and secondly to agree a common purpose or set of goals. Just who is part of this team? Are there groups that have a core function but which are often left out of team activity? These may be staff who have a different employer (perhaps a voluntary agency or the local authority) or who have different working hours or patterns which make them partially or completely invisible,[9] or perhaps people whose function may be core for patients and service users but peripheral as far as professionals are concerned. The group for whom this is often true in 'traditional' primary healthcare teams is reception staff – yet their inclusion in team discussions, rather than through the practice manager as proxy, has the potential to pay dividends.[10]

Agreeing goals, objectives and plans is also a vital part of creating a coherent team. With the advent of practice learning plans, practice accreditation and other quality-related initiatives, such developments are by no means as uncommon as they once were in traditional primary healthcare. The practice mission statements and strategies that were unusual when described by Freake and van Zwanenberg[11] have now become much more commonplace. However, similar work needs to be done in new teams, and will often have the added difficulties (but also the potential strengths) of being negotiated across different cultures (e.g. between local authority and health service staff) and between unfamiliar individuals. Focusing on patient/client/community needs can be a helpful way forward. What are we trying to achieve for them? What should they expect to see happening to their health and well-being? What factors will facilitate or hinder us in that process? What are our individual contributions to achieving this and how might they be enhanced by working together? Can we put a time scale on any of this? The use of patient participation data and community needs analyses can also help in scene setting.

Improving and maintaining a team

Once a team is established – or for that matter when a team has been around for so long that it is stale – it is important to review from time to time how the team functions, in order to maximise effectiveness in teamwork and maintain it. There are a number of dimensions to this process. First, it is important to review how well the team (which should be redefined using the above questions in case there have been any changes) is achieving the aims and objectives that are set out in its strategy. This will require some attention to the measurability of these goals, and the data available. If these aims and objectives have not been achieved, then it will be important to enable discussion of the reasons for this. For example, have the policy goalposts moved so that the objectives have become irrelevant or unachievable? Or was there an issue in relation to recruitment for a particular piece of work (e.g. a specialist clinic or a healthy community drop-in) which needs to be addressed? For instance, did the right team know what was expected and why? This discussion needs to take place in a spirit of enquiry and improvement, not one of blame.

A second important dimension of team effectiveness relates to the psychological well-being of the team itself. Indeed, if there are problems with this, it may surface in the discussion of obstacles to the achievement of the team's goals. If individuals are ill or stressed, they may well not deliver on their individual agendas, and may also have difficulty in engaging with others. If they feel valued and encouraged to contribute, they are more likely to deliver and engage. The team must therefore consider how it provides support to members, how it deals with conflicts (which arise in every team at some level – even if they are about who buys the tea and coffee!) and what the overall social 'climate' of the team is. Alongside this is the question of viability, particularly in the face of change. Many new or developing teams struggle with identity at first (*see* above). This can become a problem for an established team if an individual with a key function in the team moves on, and is perhaps replaced by someone whose role or function is different, or who at least perceives their function differently. If functions are not fulfilled, can the team continue? What needs to happen for the team to survive? Analytical tools such as Belbin's analysis of team roles[12,13] may be helpful in addressing such issues and identifying ways forward for the revised team.

The other key factor in improving and maintaining a team revolves around effective leadership. There are currently two widely accepted models of leadership in use. *Transactional* leaders lead in a charismatic and external goal-oriented way. This model is based largely on interview and biographical data from the leaders of major companies and organisations in the USA. In the *transformational* leadership model, the emphasis of most authors is on what the leader does for those whom he or she leads. In a study of effective public-sector leaders, middle managers from health and local government in the UK, Alimo-Metcalfe and Alban-Metcalfe[14] looked at the characteristics of such leaders as defined by their staff. They listed nine factors which their respondents identified as fundamental to an effective leader, namely genuine concern for others; political sensitivity and skills; decisiveness, determination and self-confidence; integrity, trustworthiness, honesty and openness; empowering and developing potential; being an inspirational networker and promoter; being accessible and approachable; clarifying boundaries and involving others in decisions; and encouraging critical and strategic thinking (*see* Box 17.1). These factors fit with a transformational model of leadership. The authors note that this list is broadly similar to those factors described by Greenleaf[15] as characteristic of a 'servant-leader'. When public-sector staff were asked to rate their own bosses in these areas, female bosses tended to score higher on these characteristics. Many successful transactional leaders are men. This may suggest a gender difference with regard to leadership style.

Box 17.1 Nine characteristics of effective leaders[14]

- Concern for others
- Political sensitivity and skills
- Decisiveness, determination and self-confidence
- Integrity, trustworthiness, honesty and openness
- Empowering and developing potential
- Inspirational networker and promoter
- Being accessible and approachable
- Clarifying boundaries and involving others in decisions
- Encouraging critical and strategic thinking

Moving forward

Whether a team working in and around community and primary healthcare is new or old, a number of factors are important in moving the team forward as a functioning entity. It is important to pinpoint who the local leaders are, and to empower them to facilitate change among their networks and teams. Successful models should be highlighted and information shared. It is also important to work with primary care trusts, local authorities and other organisations which form the broader context of the team. For some teams, particularly those which function at an interface (e.g. in intermediate care or Sure Start), it will be important to promote dialogue across different units or settings. Information systems must be robust enough to provide the data required for review when this is needed. Educators will also need to play a part, developing dialogues on appropriate curricula, responsive accreditation systems and suitable standards, and creating opportunities for learning about effective teamworking before and after qualification. Research, too, will be required, to describe practice, including innovation, clearly and accurately and to identify what really makes a difference. Teamwork is most likely to thrive when it is addressing clearly identified outcomes – especially perhaps inequalities – and when its focus is on making a concrete, measurable difference to individuals and communities.

Conclusions

The idea of the primary healthcare team has been established for decades. The ever-moving policy context of health and social care indicates that teams in the future may be rather different to those in the past, combining greater specialisation and delegation, new roles and more patient involvement. Primary healthcare teams will need to ensure that they are capable not only of working together effectively, but also of responding flexibly to change. In this chapter I have sketched out some of the advantages of collaboration and teamwork, and some of the reasons why teams and groups fail to deliver improved outcomes, or even do worse. I have suggested that in the current context an increasing number of new and reformulated teams are likely to be formed. These will need to be nurtured, and the environment and leadership within them must be facilitative. Some of the most crucial elements for developing a team will be first to develop a team identity and secondly to agree a common purpose or goals. For established teams it will be important to review how the team functions, in order to maximise and maintain effectiveness in teamwork. A key factor in team maintenance and function revolves around effective leadership. Some key elements of effective leadership have been outlined. Teamwork in community and primary care is most likely to thrive when it addresses clear outcomes and when its intention is to make a concrete, measurable difference to individuals and communities.

Practical points

- There has been confusion about who belongs to the primary healthcare team.
- An ageing workforce means that new ways of working will be needed in the future.
- Good teamwork leads to better decision making and an awareness of what works (and what does not).
- Teams need clear vision and effective leadership.
- Teams thrive where goals are clear and the focus is on making a difference to individuals and communities.

References

1 Standing Medical Advisory Committee and Standing Nursing and Midwifery Advisory Committee (1981) *The Primary Health Care Team: report of a joint working group (Harding Committee).* HMSO, London.

2 World Health Organization (1948) *The Constitution of the World Health Organization.* World Health Organization, Geneva.

3 Twigg J and Atkin K (1994) *Carers Perceived: policy and practice in informal care.* Open University Press, Buckingham.

4 Twigg J (2000) Carework as a form of bodywork. *Ageing Soc.* **20**: 389–411.

5 Wiles J (2003) Daily geographies of caregivers: mobility, routine, scale. *Soc Sci Med.* **57**(7): 1307–25.

6 West MA and Poulton BC (1997) Primary health care teams: in a league of their own. In: P Pearson and J Spencer (eds) *Promoting Teamwork in Primary Care: a research-based approach.* Arnold, London.

7 Department of Health (2002) *Shifting the Balance of Power.* Department of Health, London.

8 Usherwood T, Long S and Joesbury H (1997) The changing composition of primary health care teams. In: P Pearson and J Spencer (eds) *Promoting Teamwork in Primary Care: a research-based approach.* Arnold, London.

9 Pearson P (1997) Evaluating teambuilding. In: P Pearson and J Spencer (eds) *Promoting Teamwork in Primary Care: a research-based approach.* Arnold, London.

10 Gallagher M (2003) *Access to General Practice: a qualitative study of appointment making in general practice.* MD thesis. University of Newcastle upon Tyne, Newcastle upon Tyne.

11 Freake D and van Zwanenberg T (1997) The Practice Manifesto – a vehicle for promoting teamwork? In: P Pearson and J Spencer (eds) *Promoting Teamwork in Primary Care: a research-based approach.* Arnold, London.

12 Belbin RM (1981) *Management Teams: why they succeed or fail.* Heinemann, London.

13 Belbin RM (1996) *Team Roles at Work.* Butterworth-Heinemann, Oxford.

14 Alimo-Metcalfe B and Alban-Metcalfe RJ (2001) The development of a new Transformational Leadership Questionnaire. *J Occup Organiz Psychol.* **74**: 1–27.

15 Greenleaf RK (1996) *On Becoming a Servant-Leader.* Jossey-Bass, New York.

PART 3

Exploring the future

CHAPTER 18

Educating the coming generation

John Spencer

Medical education is a reflection of medical practice; it is not the education that will change the practitioners, but reformed practice that will redesign medical education.

George Silver (1983)

This chapter explains how the clinical governance agenda is already present within the undergraduate and training curriculum. It highlights the need to embody clinical governance in all aspects of the student's experience, and introduces the concept of curricular governance.

The background

It is self-evident that health professions in training should be prepared for the challenges of future practice – as far, that is, as such challenges can be anticipated. Indeed, much has been written about the need to ensure that all basic professional training takes account of both the emerging role of the doctor- or nurse-to-be and the realities of everyday practice, and that such education is relevant to the changing needs and expectations of society.[1,2]

Equally, implementing clinical governance and making it work will remain one of the major challenges facing healthcare professionals in the UK for the foreseeable future. Such a task has important implications for those involved in the basic education of doctors, nurses and other professions allied to medicine. Although in the various policy documents much has been written about the educational implications of clinical governance for *established* practitioners, conspicuous by their absence are any substantive references to the implications for the basic education of health professionals. When the issue *is* mentioned, universities are criticised for having neither 'adopted the new quality agenda' nor helped learners develop the skills of 'knowledge management'.[3]

Undergraduate medical education in the UK has undergone radical change in the last decade, largely in response to and guided by the recommendations of the

General Medical Council (GMC) in its influential document *Tomorrow's Doctors*, first published in 1993.[4] This identified the need to produce doctors whose attitude to both medicine and learning would equip them for lifelong professional careers. Thus where lifelong learning becomes the main aim of the undergraduate course, what is required (among other things) is a reduction in the factual burden of curricula, and the promotion of the capacity for self-education, reduction in error, evaluation of evidence and critical thinking. Within a culture of lifelong learning must also come the ability to forget, thereby putting aside ways of thinking and acting that have become outmoded. *Tomorrow's Doctors* was updated in 2002.[5]

Implicit in these recommendations, and made explicit in other GMC publications, notably *Good Medical Practice*,[6] was the nature of the contract between the medical profession and society. Issues such as the need for high moral and ethical standards, the importance of keeping up to date, the duty to protect all patients and the importance of working in teams are all highlighted. *Good Medical Practice* is not only a framework for appraisal, revalidation and assessment of poor performance for *established* practitioners, but also has relevance for basic education. The key elements are listed in Box 18.1.

Box 18.1   Key elements of good medical practice

- Good clinical care
- Maintaining good medical practice
- Relationships with patients
- Working with colleagues
- Teaching and training
- Probity
- Health and conduct

From *Good Medical Practice*[6]

Similar changes have taken place in nurse education.[7]

Another major driver of change has been the increasing prominence given to education about professionalism in undergraduate courses, in the context of a wider debate about the nature and components of professionalism itself. This has taken place at a time when the medical profession has come under increasing fire – for failing to self-regulate, for turning a blind eye to unethical or incompetent practice, and for continuing paternalism and poor communication – all this in an era when what the public wants is greater accountability, partnership and respect.[8] For example, in 2002, following international collaboration, the *Charter for Medical Professionalism* was published simultaneously in two prestigious medical journals, one on each side of the Atlantic.[9,10]

The Charter outlined three principles to which all medical professionals should aspire (the primacy of patients' welfare, respect for their autonomy and the promotion of social justice), and a set of responsibilities to which they should be committed (*see* Box 18.2). It can be seen that many of these areas are pertinent to the clinical governance agenda. The Charter aims to promote 'an action agenda, universal in scope and purpose', including education about professionalism.

Box 18.2   A set of professional responsibilities to which doctors should be committed

- Professional competence
- Patient confidentiality
- Maintaining appropriate relationships with patients
- Improving the quality of care
- Improving access to care
- Just distribution of finite resources
- Scientific knowledge
- Maintaining trust
- Professional responsibilities

From the *Charter for Medical Professionalism*[9,10]

Implications for the education of healthcare practitioners

The implications of clinical governance for the education of healthcare practitioners have been discussed in the literature. The second edition of *Tomorrow's Doctors* actually states that 'the graduate must be aware of current developments and guiding principles in the NHS – for example, systems of quality assurance such as clinical governance'.[5] An editorial that concerned itself as much with the education of nurses and other healthcare professionals as with the education of doctors highlighted several key issues[11] (*see* Box 18.3).

Box 18.3   Key issues for medical educators in relation to clinical governance

- Ensure the acquisition of requisite skills and understanding
- Introduce the concept of clinical governance early on
- Apply the principles of clinical governance to educational activities
- Promote the values that underpin clinical governance

From Morrison and Buckley[11]

First, learners need to acquire the necessary understanding and skills if they are to utilise such tools as clinical audit, critical appraisal and risk assessment. Secondly, the concept of clinical governance should be introduced from the beginning, and remain as a continuous theme in curricula. Thirdly, educators must be prepared to practise what they preach, and to apply the principles of clinical governance to their own educational activities. Finally, and perhaps most important of all, it is necessary to promote the values that underpin the concept of clinical governance. To this list of issues could also be added the need to develop appropriate skills and attitudes in relation to teamwork, and the ability to use the principles of management effectively.

Other authors have highlighted similar issues,[12] emphasising the need to create a safe learning environment and to promote the values and skills of self and peer audit, constructive feedback and reflective practice. Suggestions for teaching about clinical governance have been made. These are summarised in Box 18.4.

Box 18.4 Suggestions for teaching about clinical governance

- Use simple maps and models
- Put clinical governance in a historical context
- Identify individual elements and use clinical examples
- Define learning outcomes
- Teach about change management
- Teach the skills of appraisal and feedback
- Promote reflection
- Teach the principles and limitations of evidence-based practice
- Foster team development
- Encourage evaluation

Adapted from Houghton and Wall[12]

The current situation
Gaining understanding and learning skills

Many of the component activities of clinical governance are already being addressed in undergraduate curricula and pre-registration courses. For instance, innovative models for teaching and learning about clinical audit have been described – for example, where medical students undertake audit projects during clinical attachments in general practice. These brief courses are generally highly valued by students, and involvement in them also appears to be beneficial for GP tutors and patients alike.[13,14] Similar outcomes have been described in surgical settings.[15]

Models and methods are available for teaching the skills of critical appraisal and evidence-based practice[16] and for learning about medical informatics, encompassing a broad range of topics, including clinical information systems, medical record keeping, decision making and decision support, and the use of guidelines.[17] However, as with all areas of innovation, there is a need for rigorous evaluation.[18]

Teaching and learning about ethics and medical aspects of law are now well established in undergraduate curricula, often being taught alongside communication skills, and recommendations have been made about a 'core' curriculum for the content of such courses.[19] With ethics and the law come moral questions about life and death, rationing and being professionals in today's world. Grounding all such learning as far as possible in practice rather than in theory, and on concrete examples (ideally real cases based on the experiences of the learners), is vital. This promotes relevance, fosters integration of knowledge and motivates learners.[2,20]

Teamworking

Effective teamworking is said to promote clinical governance. Interprofessional education, whereby students from different professional backgrounds in health and social care spend time learning together, is seen as one means whereby teamworking skills might be developed.[21] The past few years have seen an increasing number of initiatives to explore the potential of interprofessional education. To date, evidence in support of its efficacy is limited. Simple descriptions of courses are more common in the literature than any evidence of their effectiveness, and evaluations of benefits beyond the short term have been marred by methodological problems.[22,23]

Nonetheless, there have been some studies of interprofessional education (both in the UK and elsewhere) that have demonstrated increased mutual understanding and respect, through the identification of 'common values, knowledge and skills across professions and work settings and creating a shared philosophy of care',[22] with more positive attitudes towards the importance of multidisciplinary teamwork and communication as a result.[24] Despite the lack of evidence so far, intuitively it seems the right thing to encourage shared learning, with the potential to influence the development of the practitioners of the new century, for whom new ways of working together are an inevitability.

Introducing the concept of clinical governance systematically

The increased emphasis in the curricula on skills acquisition, 'knowledge management',[3] ethical reasoning and the promotion of lifelong learning, as well as on pastoral and personal development and the development of professionalism, has led to the development in many medical schools of courses that draw such themes together into a coherent curricular structure. These courses start early and run through the whole curriculum, interweaving – where appropriate – with teaching and learning in the basic and clinical sciences. This integration provides an ideal vehicle for introducing concepts of clinical governance. At the same time, the so-called 'man in society'-type courses[4] (which usually cover human development, aspects of sociology and psychology that are relevant to health, illness and disease, and so on) have also been introduced, alongside an increased emphasis on population medicine.

Such courses are relatively new phenomena, and appropriate models and methods are still evolving.[25] However, whatever the challenges, the need for professional development to become part of the core undergraduate curriculum, as opposed to a 'bolt-on' extra, is widely accepted.[26]

An example from the 2001 curriculum at the Newcastle–Durham Medical School is shown in Box 18.5. This 'Personal and Professional Development Strand' is introduced in the first week of the medical course, and is set in the context of the GMC's *Good Medical Practice*.[6]

A broad view of communication skills is taken, including not only doctor–patient communication but also communication with colleagues, written and presentation skills, and group and teamworking skills. A patient-centred approach to communication is promoted, whereby the patient's illness experience is elicited and incorporated into clinical decisions in order to achieve a shared understanding.[27]

Box 18.5 The 'Personal and Professional Development Strand' at Newcastle–Durham Medical School (2001 curriculum)

- Starts in first year and runs as a vertical theme throughout the five-year curriculum
- Integrates with teaching and learning in basic and clinical sciences
- Is assessed where appropriate

Themes
- Communication skills
- Clinical skills
- Ethics
- Methods of enquiry
- Clinical reasoning
- Context of care
- Self-care (including study skills support and pastoral support)

'Methods of enquiry' covers a wide range of skills related to 'knowledge management', including critical appraisal and evidence-based medicine, communication and information technology and searching skills, research methods and statistics, and decision making. 'Context of care' emphasises that healthcare is delivered in a multiplicity of settings by a wide variety of healthcare professionals, each professional group having its own internal 'culture'. That culture influences the organisation of teams, relationships and even the way in which care is ultimately delivered.

Professional codes of practice are explored alongside basic principles in the 'ethics' component. Here teaching focuses as much on the ethical challenges that face practitioners in everyday practice (e.g. dealing with error, seeking informed consent) as it does on the 'big issues' (e.g. euthanasia, reproductive technology).

The 'self-care' component addresses personal development through both academic and pastoral support. This area has been somewhat neglected in medical education in the past. In view of the high levels of stress and maladaptive behaviours reported by medical students,[28] and the influence that this might have on subsequent morale and performance, this neglect needs to be addressed.

The development of reflective abilities is highly pertinent to clinical governance. Promotion of reflective practice[29] and of self-awareness is already well developed in nurse education,[30] and is an emerging theme in undergraduate medical curricula.[31]

Practising what we preach: curricular governance

In parallel with the development and implementation of new courses in medical schools, there has been something of a cultural change in the way in which curricula are managed. This has come about partly in response to increasing concern about quality issues, with demands for greater accountability, and partly as an inevitable consequence of moving towards more innovative educational approaches. Curriculum design, implementation and management have become more strategic, underpinned by recognition of the fact that underlying systems are as important as course content in the delivery of high-quality teaching and learning.

Curriculum governance has been described as 'a system through which teaching institutions and individual teachers are accountable for continuously improving the quality of their course and safeguarding high standards of teaching by creating an environment in which excellence in teaching and learning will flourish' (J Bligh, personal communication) and, like its clinical counterpart, it resonates with corporate governance. Essential components of curriculum governance must therefore include strong and transparent management systems, rigorous and systematic evaluation of courses, and staff development.[32,33]

Student involvement is a key element of curriculum governance, and plays an important part in the process of quality management and enhancement. Here students assume a role equivalent to that of patients in the context of clinical governance, and for them this involvement creates a sense of ownership and partnership, and may even improve motivation.[34,35] Many medical schools have been particularly innovative in involving students in the curriculum (e.g. Liverpool, with its student parliament, and Manchester, through student involvement in staff development.[36,37]

Promoting appropriate values

Clinical governance is as much about an attitude of mind as it is about skills and systems. Inculcation of appropriate professional attitudes and values has assumed prominence in the recommendations of the bodies that govern basic and pre-registration education of healthcare professionals. For example, the GMC describes a range of attitudinal outcomes in the latest edition of *Tomorrow's Doctors*, using the framework of *Good Medical Practice*. All of them, to a greater or lesser extent, have some relevance to learning about clinical governance – for example, 'be willing to respond constructively to the outcome of appraisal, performance review and assessment.'[5]

The increased emphasis on communication should also help students to adopt a clinical method that is patient centred (rather than the traditional paternalistic approach) – one that fosters a genuine partnership between healthcare professional and patient.[27] Facilitating the development of attitudes is one thing. However, if the acquisition of such attitudes is not assessed in some way, it will not be given a high priority by students. Similarly, if students do not see clinical governance 'in action' during their clinical attachments, the impact of the teaching and learning will be diluted considerably. The concept of the 'hidden curriculum' is useful in this context. A curriculum can be thought of as consisting of three elements, namely 'the curriculum on paper' (what is intended or what it is hoped the course will achieve), 'the curriculum in action' (what is delivered on the day) and 'the curriculum the student experiences'. The latter can be very different both from what is intended and from what actually happens. The relationship between these three curricula is shown in Figure 18.1.

The part of the curriculum that is neither explicitly intended nor formally taught is known as the 'hidden curriculum'. This was first described in the context

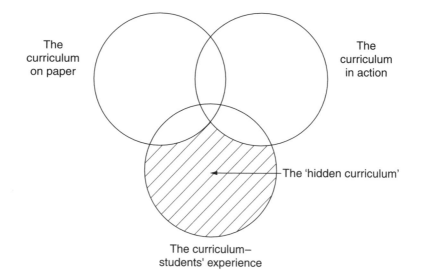

Figure 18.1 The three curricula and the hidden curriculum.

of primary school education,[38] but is a potent force in all educational settings and forms a large part of a student's learning experience. It is effectively a 'parallel' curriculum through which students learn the values, norms and expectations of an educational environment. It can be a more powerful influence than teachers might imagine (e.g. in the socialisation of students, or in determining whether students decide to study a subject based on whether it is assessed).

One cannot overestimate the effect that assessment has in driving learning, influencing both *what* students learn and *how* they learn it, quite literally 'the tail that wags the dog'. It is therefore important, with regard to teaching and learning about clinical governance, to ensure that whatever relevant areas can be appropriately assessed actually *are* assessed.

Historically, assessment of attitudes has been somewhat neglected in medical education, not least because it is a difficult and challenging area compared with assessment of skills and knowledge. A recent review of approaches to assessing professionalism concluded that although the current array of assessment instruments is rich and holds great potential, their measurement properties must be strengthened and evaluated.[39]

The role of primary care in the basic education of healthcare professionals

One trend that has been gathering momentum in healthcare education in recent years is the move to deliver more basic teaching and learning in the community. In the context of medical education in the UK, this has usually meant more experience in general practice, although increasingly a wider view of the 'community' is being taken.[22,40]

As well as learning specifically about the discipline of general practice, doctors in training are exposed to a wide range of learning opportunities,[41] including the following:

- learning about health, disease and disability in its social context, and about the environmental and social determinants of disease
- seeing the full range of presentation of health problems
- having opportunities to learn basic clinical and communication skills on relatively healthy patients
- experiencing a more holistic approach to patient care
- better integration of knowledge and understanding
- experiencing continuity of care
- learning to manage uncertainty and to handle ambiguity
- seeing multidisciplinary teamwork in action.

It has been argued that in many ways primary care is the ideal setting for educating 'tomorrow's doctors', where critical reasoning, self-awareness and reflexivity, and the ability to handle uncertainty – all of which are highly pertinent in the context of clinical governance – can be fostered.[42]

Making it happen: curricular change

Implementing curricular change is difficult. Models for managing innovation in medical education have been outlined,[43] and the process starts with the identification of potential barriers. One key barrier can be the resistance and scepticism of colleagues, who may view clinical governance as nothing more than 'a mixture of the blindingly obvious (people should lead well and work well in teams) and the unproved (clinical audit)'.[44] Other important obstacles may include chronic curriculum overload, attitudes that view any curricular content 'beyond' the strictly biomedical as superfluous (and therefore a waste of curricular time) and, of course, the thorny question of how to resource the teaching.

A relatively new approach to curriculum design and management (and thus to curricular change) which is gaining ground in a wide range of contexts in healthcare education, including undergraduate programmes, is the so-called *outcomes based approach*.[45] Here the intended outcomes of learning are expressed in a form that permits their achievement to be demonstrated and measured. In its simplest form it has three components, namely explicit statements of learning intent, which reflect the educational aims, purposes and values of the programme (e.g. 'be able to communicate effectively and sensitively with patients and their relatives'); the process by which they may be achieved; and the criteria for assessing their achievement, and at what level. Learning outcomes thus set the agenda and define what is (and by implication what is not) essential. The advantages claimed for this approach are that it makes the educational process transparent, it provides a framework for all aspects of the curriculum, and it promotes relevance.

In terms of the learning process, problem-based learning is mentioned as one approach which 'should in time improve teamworking skills'.[21] Although there is controversy over some of the benefits claimed by problem-based learning, there are many areas of practice pertinent to clinical governance where a problem-based approach could make a significant contribution – not least in the development, enhancement and retention of self-directed learning skills.[46] Other curricular approaches, such as 'guided discovery learning', which combine innovative methods with the best of traditional modes, may also be just as effective in promoting self-directed learning.[47]

Conclusions

This chapter has argued that most of the basic building blocks for learning about clinical governance are already in place in medical undergraduate curricula. Furthermore, a culture is evolving in which *curriculum* governance can provide an analogous framework in which students learn about the basic principles of governance itself. This process needs to be extended to the basic training of all healthcare practitioners, and should be seen as a normal part of the curriculum – properly assessed and resourced. Equally, only when clinical governance is seen in action in normal everyday practice will it be taken seriously by all those in training. Failure to do so will have profound implications for the way in which tomorrow's healthcare professionals do their job.

Practical points

- The training of future practitioners requires flexibility and vision.
- Undergraduate curricula already address much of the clinical governance agenda.
- Learning about ethics, teamworking, communication with patients and coping with stress is vital for all.
- Curricular governance provides insights for clinical governance.
- The best way to learn is to experience clinical governance in action.

References

1 Calman K (1994) The profession of medicine. *BMJ*. **309**: 1140–3.
2 Chastonay P, Brenner E, Peel S and Guilbert J-J (1996) The need for more efficacy and relevance in medical education. *Med Educ*. **30**: 235–8.
3 Donaldson LJ and Muir Gray JA (1998) Clinical governance: a quality duty for health organisations. *Qual Health Care*. **7 (Supplement 1)**: S37–44.
4 General Medical Council (1993) *Tomorrow's Doctors: recommendations on undergraduate medical education*. General Medical Council, London.
5 General Medical Council (2002) *Tomorrow's Doctors*. General Medical Council, London.
6 General Medical Council (1995) *Good Medical Practice*. General Medical Council, London.
7 www.nmc-uk.org/cms/content/home/ (accessed June 2003).

8 Spencer J (2003) Teaching tomorrow's doctors. In: J Harrison, R Innes and T van Zwanenberg (eds) *Rebuilding Trust in Healthcare*. Radcliffe Medical Press, Oxford.

9 Medical Professionalism Project (2002) Medical professionalism in the new millennium: a physician's charter. *Lancet*. **359**: 520–2.

10 American Board of Internal Medicine (2002) Medical professionalism in the new millennium: a physician's charter. *Ann Intern Med*. **136**: 243–6.

11 Morrison J and Buckley G (1999) Clinical governance – implications for medical education. *Med Educ*. **33**: 162–4.

12 Houghton G and Wall D (2001) Twelve tips on teaching about clinical governance. *Med Teacher*. **22**: 145–53.

13 Morrison JM and Sullivan FM (1997) Audit in general practice: educating medical students. *Med Educ*. **31**: 128–31.

14 Howe AC and Purkiss V (1998) Resourcing innovative teaching of audit – models, methods and MAAGs. *Med Educ*. **32**: 607–12.

15 Rudkin GE, O'Driscoll MCE and Lind R (1999) Can medical students contribute to quality assurance programmes in day surgery? *Med Educ*. **33**: 509–14.

16 Sackett DL, Strauss S, Richardson S, Rosenberg W and Haynes RB (2000) *Evidence-Based Medicine: how to practice and teach EBM* (2e). Churchill Livingstone, London.

17 Purves I (1995) *Integrating Medical Informatics Into the Medical Undergraduate Curriculum: a theoretical overview using Newcastle University as a template*. Sowerby Unit for Primary Care Informatics, Newcastle upon Tyne.

18 Sullivan F (1999) Informatics in medical education. *Med Teacher*. **21**: 541–2.

19 Ashcroft R, Baron D, Benatar S *et al*. (1998) Teaching medical ethics and law within medical education: a model for the UK core curriculum. *J Med Ethics*. **24**: 188–92.

20 Coles C (1997) How students learn: the process of learning. In: B Jolly and L Rees (eds) *Medical Education in the Millennium*. Oxford Medical Publications, Oxford.

21 Scally G and Donaldson LJ (1998) Clinical governance and the drive for quality improvement in the new NHS in England. *BMJ*. **317**: 61–5.

22 Boaden N and Bligh J (1999) *Community-Based Medical Education*. Arnold, London.

23 Barr H (2002) *Inter-Professional Education: today, yesterday and tomorrow*. Learning and Teaching Support Network for Health Sciences and Practice, London.

24 Carpenter J (1995) Doctors and nurses: stereotypes and stereotype change in interprofessional education. *J Interprof Care*. **9**: 151–61.

25 Gordon J (2003) Fostering students' personal and professional development in medicine: a new framework for PPD. *Med Educ*. **37**: 341–9.

26 Spencer J (2003) Teaching about professionalism. *Med Educ* **37**: 287.

27 Stewart M, Belle Brown J, Wayne Weston W, McWhinney IR, McWilliam CL and Freeman TR (2003) *Patient-Centered Medicine: transforming the clinical method* (2e). Radcliffe Medical Press, Oxford.

28 Webb E, Ashton H, Kelly P and Kamali F (1998) An update on British medical students' lifestyles. *Med Educ*. **32**: 325–31.

29 Westberg J and Jason H (2001) *Fostering Reflection and Providing Feedback: helping others learn from experience*. Springer Publishing Company, New York.

30 Richardson G and Maltby H (1995) Reflection on practice: enhancing student learning. *J Adv Nurs*. **22**: 235–42.

31 Novack DH, Suchman AL, Clark W, Epstein RM, Najberg E and Kaplan C (1997) Calibrating the physician. Personal awareness and effective patient care. *JAMA*. **278**: 502–9.

32 Elton L (1997) Staff development and the quality of teaching. In: B Jolly and L Rees (eds) *Medical Education in the Millennium*. Oxford Medical Publications, Oxford.

33 Wilkes M and Bligh J (1999) Evaluating educational interventions. *BMJ*. **318**: 1269–72.

34 Prince CJAH and Visser K (1997) The student as quality controller. In: AJJA Scherpbier, CPM van der Vleuten, JJ Rethans and AFW van der Steed (eds) *Advances in Medical Education*. Kluwer Academic Publishers, Dordrecht.

35 Visser K, Prince CJ, Scherpbier AJ *et al*. (1998) Student participation in educational management and organisation. *Med Teacher*. **20**: 451–4.

36 www.liv.ac.uk/FacultyMedicine/vrc/ugcourse.html (accessed June 2003).

37 Duffy KA and O'Neill PA (2003) Involving medical students in staff development activities. *Med Teacher*. **25**: 191–4.

38 Jackson P (1996) The student's world. *Elementary School J*. **66**: 353.

39 Arnold L (2002) Assessing professional behaviour: yesterday, today and tomorrow. *Acad Med*. **77**: 502–15.

40 Seabrook M, Lempp H and Woodfield S (1998) *Extending Community Involvement in Medical Education: a guide*. King's Undergraduate Medical Education in the Community, London.

41 Spencer J (2002) What can undergraduate education offer general practice? In: J Harrison and T van Zwanenberg (eds) *GP Tomorrow*. Radcliffe Medical Press, Oxford.

42 Oswald NTA (1996) Doctors for the twenty-first century: the contribution primary medical care could make. *Educ Health*. **9**: 37–44.

43 Gale R and Grant J (1990) *Managing Change in a Medical Context: guidelines for action*. The Joint Centre, London.

44 Goodman N (1998) Clinical governance. *BMJ*. **317**: 1725–7.

45 Spencer J and Jordan R (2001) Educational outcomes and leadership to meet the needs of modern health care. *Qual Health Care*. **10 (Supplement II)**: ii38–45.

46 Finucane PM, Johnson SM and Prideaux DJ (1998) Problem-based learning: its rationale and efficacy. *Med J Aust*. **168**: 445–8.

47 Spencer JA and Jordan RK (1999) Learner-centred approaches in medical education. *BMJ*. **318**: 1280–3.

CHAPTER 19

The end of certainty: professionalism revisited

Jamie Harrison and Robert Innes

All professions are conspiracies against the laity.

George Bernard Shaw

> This chapter explores what it means to be health service professionals for today. After all, what is 'health'? And how, against a background of rising expectations of healthcare, can clinical governance help to define and enhance the future 'bargain' between the practitioner and the patient?

The right to health

According to the World Health Organization (WHO), the possession of health is a basic human right.[1] Since the eighteenth century, the question of whether individuals have a 'right to health' has been keenly debated. Indeed, the French Revolutionary 'Health Committee of the National Constituent Assembly' formally supported the idea that health was a natural right to which all citizens were entitled, asserting that if the role of government was to protect natural rights, then public health was a duty of the state. More recently, the WHO itself has taken up the campaign of 'Health for all by the year 2000'.

Yet governments struggle to make sense of health planning and the provision of health services. The power of consumerist electorates has driven them into defensive mode as they try to keep up with burgeoning expectations. Thomas Osborne summarises the position as follows:

> From the idea that it is the duty of a government to secure the well-being of the population, it is not such a large step – and a nice instance, besides, of the strategic 'reversibility' of power relations – to the parallel idea that it is a right of the population to be provided with health and well-being.[2]

To be required to guarantee health and well-being to the population is, of course, quite different from having to provide access to essential healthcare to individuals and families.[3] Equally, using the language of rights may be mistaken. Rights are, in principle, capable of being asserted against some body (individual or corporate). However, individuals are primarily responsible for their own health. And how can a person assert a right against him- or herself?

Defining health

> Health is one of a number of words which are constantly in use and which are so rich in meaning that they cannot be explained fully without involving controversy.[4]

The definition of the word 'health' itself is difficult. As soon as it comes into view, health escapes over the horizon to reposition itself. This remains a nightmare as much for policy makers as for practitioners. What was accepted as a reasonable state of health a few years ago (the odd back pain, an occasional cold and intermittent bouts of indigestion) may now be seen as deeply unhealthy. Even one (however tragic) death from meningitis is apparently unacceptable. Being healthy seems to be an increasingly unattainable goal. Osborne goes on to quote philosopher Georges Canguilhem's provocative point:

> Health is essentially a negative state rather than a positive one; when one is healthy one is oblivious of the issue of health or ill-health as a problem.[2]

For Canguilhem, health is something we cannot know positively – or at least we can only know it, so to speak, in its absence. This makes defining health even more difficult.

Some definitions of health describe an ideal state of being – an *end* in itself – which all might attain (i.e. perfect health). Others delineate health pragmatically, as the *means* that enables people to live a proper life (i.e. the vehicle to self-realisation). The WHO definition of health as 'a state of complete physical, mental and social well-being, not merely the absence of disease and handicap'[1] is an example of the former approach. Idealised definitions, while laying down markers for action, place the proffered ideal state outside the realm of real people.

The risk of such universal, perfectionist approaches is that they undermine the efforts of those who set out on the quest to establish health. Who would not give up as the impossibility of the task became apparent? And what patient could possibly experience such a Utopian state for any length of time? The claims made by ordinary citizens who might embrace such a definition simply could not be fulfilled by any government or health service. The result could be that the power of medicine would be overestimated, and that permanently excessive demands would be made of doctors.

The second approach is illustrated by the writings of German theologian Jürgen Moltmann. For Moltmann, health is 'the strength to be human'.[5] Here the intention is to portray health as the means by which human beings achieve their full potential. Obstacles to health – whether they be biological, environmental, societal, familial or personal – must be faced and overcome. 'Strength' is not to be equated with strong muscles or performance on a treadmill test. Rather it is that person-specific quality which is utilised by individuals as they work towards living a fulfilled life. David Seedhouse values the way in which the humanist Katherine Mansfield puts it:

> By health I mean the power to live a full adult, living, breathing, life …
> I want to be all that I am capable of becoming.

Seedhouse goes on to talk of health as an essentially enabling quality. It is about providing 'appropriate foundations for achieving potential'.[4]

Rights, responsibilities and clinical governance

To be fair to the World Health Organization, the Alma-Ata Declaration speaks of both rights and responsibilities:

> For their part, the people will learn to identify their real health needs and to become involved in and promote community action for health. Thus, society will come to realise that health is not only the right of all but also the *responsibility* of all, and the members of the health professions, too, will find their proper role.[3]

Yet encouraging individuals to assume the primary responsibility for their own health is notoriously difficult. Alastair Campbell notes the critique of René Dubos:

> To ward off disease or recover health, man as a rule finds it easier to depend on healers than to attempt the more difficult task of living wisely.[6]

The challenge for clinical governance is clear. How do you set about improving service quality and safeguarding high standards without at the same time encouraging a culture of dependency and false expectation among patients? (This has been a criticism of government charters.) For to live out one's full humanity, with all of its problems, will involve negotiation between what is possible, what is desirable and what should be left well alone.

Promising an excellent service could set the ideal so high that it does no one any favours – confusing the offer of health with that of happiness. One of our most urgent requirements is to find a more adequate definition of health, while at the same time making it much clearer to the public imagination the strictly limited role that medical intervention has in securing health.

This is a difficult theme as it contradicts the popular model of modern medicine, where every promise can be fulfilled – even, perhaps, making people happy.[7] The perceived shortcomings of technological medicine (for all its successes) raise the question of who is to blame when things go wrong, or at least do not follow the perfect plan. For in an individualistic, postmodern world someone or something must be to blame. As Campbell writes:

> The practice of medicine is all too easily destroyed by the inappropriate expectations of patients and by the false pretensions of doctors.[6]

Litigation

We are all conscious of the need to address malpractice and under-performance. Yet society must ask itself at what point pursuing practitioners to maximise their clinical performance becomes counter-productive. For instance, it has become increasingly hard to find an obstetrician in some parts of the USA, such has become the cost of indemnity insurance and the risk of litigation. The desire for a perfect baby has its difficulties.

> American attitudes have exacerbated the situation. There, consumer-ism dominates medicine. With the right treatment, doctor and hospital, nothing need ever kill you. If anything goes wrong, you – or your relatives – can always sue.[8]

So what does constitute a reasonable, adequate or acceptable level of clinical service? If only the best is good enough, and clinical governance expects high standards to be safeguarded and quality to be continuously improved, then the highest performing unit for every subspecialty would need to be identified and its level of performance noted.

But would all other similar but less effective units be required to close? One criticism of the Bristol cardiac surgery unit was that the performance of the surgeons was not up to that of, say, the units at Great Ormond Street. Should all cases, then, go to the national centre (in this case in London) where the team has the exclusive expertise?

An increase in litigation may reflect a loss of trust in the promises that modernity (especially modern scientific medicine) seemed to be making. At the same time, Utopian notions of health involve a heightened desire for the risk-free (perfect) existence. Yet most people's experience is of a progressive awareness of their own mortality. This goes with the fragmentation of the support structures of life. How then can we hold on to the wonder which is life itself?

> From one perspective indeed a human life is not of much significance – birth, growth, death in the space of a few years. Yet that being is capable of loving and being loved, and in consequence is of great value.[9]

The practitioner's task does not come to an end when the resources of curative medical science are exhausted. He or she is required to exercise the love and care of a friend, being with and affirming the one who is dying.[10]

From regulation to risk society

Allied to this shift in sensibility from trust towards litigation has been the move from a regulated society to one that is characterised by risk.[11] The old nationalised bureaucracies (public utilities, rail and air travel, etc.) have been privatised. Deregulation has been the trend of the last decade. With this deregulation comes uncertainty, flexibility and risk. Will it work? Who will pick up the pieces if it does not? Will the 'nanny state' still be there when we need her?

At the same time, the general public has been exposed to a catalogue of looming disasters, from 'decimation' through HIV/AIDS, new variant CJD and 'flesh-eating bugs' to the sudden overwhelming threat of meningitis. Therefore it is not surprising that there is disquiet when people hear of doctors failing in the simpler tasks. Governments worry, too:

> A risk society, based on deregulation and devolution, often requires more subtle and systematic forms of control. For example, the state is forced to create regulatory systems of quality control where public utilities have been privatised.[12]

The formation of primary care groups opens up the spectre of small, flexible, budget-limited healthcare organisations being required to manage the risks present in their local health domains. What then is the role of the professional in such an organisation, which is increasingly being asked to provide a uniformly high standard of service to the general public? And all of this is happening at a time when the medical profession is itself under severe scrutiny by itself, the public and the media alike.[13,14]

The nature of professionalism

Much has been made recently of the moves towards revalidation by the GMC and the potential powers of the Commission for Health Improvement. To what extent should the professionals, especially those in a publicly funded service, be directly supervised and to what extent should they be left to their own monitoring of performance? To what extent should peers be encouraged to participate in performance review? Will they be objective or will they collude? And what of patients – the 'consumers' of the 'product'? In what ways should they be involved?

For at a fundamental level, an understanding of what goes on between the patient and the doctor or nurse must be shared and agreed. What is this so-called 'bargain' that must be struck between them? How does this relationship differ from that between customer and salesman, or between master and servant? Does it matter whether you are in a public or private organisation? Are health professionals contracted or covenanted to their patients? In what ways do patients behave as good citizens, with virtues and responsibilities (*see* Box 19.1)?

Box 19.1   Characteristics of citizens and professionals

The good citizen
- Expert on own body
- Expects good care
- Responsible
- Realistic
- Informed
- Experiences whole of life
- Accepts a team response
- Assumes effective regulation
- Respects professionalism

The professional
- Humble
- Consistently competent
- Responsive
- Accessible
- Keeps up to date
- Flexible
- Teamworker
- Self-regulating
- Follows code of conduct

Partnership between professional carers and those for whom they care points one way forward. Yet all partnerships risk exploitative relationships, either in terms of unequal power relationships or in terms of expecting too much of the other. As one young doctor has commented, 'doctors offered everything on the basis that patients would not ask too much'.[15] For too long, doctors in particular seemed to hold the upper hand. Are patients now asking for more? Ken Jarrold puts this issue into stark relief:

> Although we often only pay lip service to their existence, patients and carers are at the heart of the NHS. Although events at Bristol and in many other places may give the impression that the NHS exists for the benefit of professional staff – it does not. The NHS exists for patients and carers.[16]

A culture of professionalism and partnership must be fostered. Without it, patients really do just become objects of the financial machine, viewed either as 'consumers' or as 'sources of income'. However, in an increasingly suspicious and fragmented age, how can such a culture be sustained (*see* Box 19.2)?

Box 19.2 Attitudes that affect the citizen–professional relationship

Negatively
- Criticism
- Contempt
- Defensiveness
- Withdrawal

Positively
- Encouragement
- Openness
- Respect
- Engagement

Power, transparency and interpretation

If indeed patients are to work in partnership with their professional carers, then transparency and honesty are necessary on both sides. In an increasingly complex technological age, where information overloads the consultation and both doctor and patient can become more and more bewildered by facts and opinions, shared understandings take on a new significance.

Ian Purves writes of doctor–patient interactions in which 'the computer needs to become the third member in the triadic relationship of the consultation.'[17] The computer offers up 'information' which the doctor seeks to integrate into the patient's story. Informed, shared decision making follows, as narrative and objective clinical data are synthesised. This 'hermeneutical'[18] process can then lead to a writing of the story for the future, after the consultation. In this way, rights are replaced by partnerships or covenanted relationships, and both the patient and the health professional are seen as bearing equal responsibility in the attempt to produce – or maintain – an acceptable state of health and well-being.

Hermeneutics and healing

Thus questions emerge for both patients and practitioners. Is medicine a science or an art? It is a technique or a practice? Our contemporary culture emphasises the predominance of science – the medical world itself according most prestige to the technical work of specialists, rather than to the personal role of generalists.

However, a moment's reflection makes it obvious that medicine is not pure science. William Osler called medicine 'a science of uncertainty and an art of probability.'[19] Illness is a subjective state. As such, it is not exactly reducible to objective measurements. A patient walks into the surgery and the doctor asks 'How are you?' This question cannot be answered in the language of pure science. Or at least anyone who tries to answer it in this way has misunderstood the way in which the language works.

The healer's art begins with listening to the patient's self-description, with sufficient attentiveness and warmth to gain the patient's trust for the whole story. Here begins the work of clinical wisdom, for what follows is the beginning of an interpretation about what is going on in the patient's life and body. Without this initial way into the patient's story, all that should follow – the early judgement, working diagnosis and subsequent prognosis – is lost.

Obviously science has a vital place, but scientific reasoning does not of itself lead to action. The science must be integrated into the biography of the particular patient (the narrative), and vice versa, so that deductive and practical reasoning lead to wise action – what Ian Purves has called 'the art and the science of the art of medicine.'[17]

Clinical governance and the bargain with patients

The peculiar mix of art and science appears to be paradoxical. Patients on the one hand demand rationality, but on the other hand they hate the idea that they can be rationalised (and in addition they fear that services to them may be rationed). No one wants to be thought of as a mere machine.

Successful medicine involves the restoration of wholeness, or at least fosters the patient's own strength to be human – co-operating with the body's own natural healing processes with minimal interference. Gadamer gives the illustration of tree-cutting with a two-handed saw – two people working together harmoniously. However, if one person applies too much force, the blade will jam.[20]

This analogy of the two-handed saw also applies to the bargain between patients and practitioners. For clinical governance to work effectively, this relationship must be both transparent and co-operative in nature. It is no longer permissible to claim a professional monopoly of power in the healing process. Patients have the right to equal partnership, and NHS organisations are accountable to them. They deserve high standards – indeed excellence of care, as the governance definition puts it.

Yet patients already recognise that doctors and nurses are under severe pressure at work. They do not wish to see this pressure increase, and are willing to share the burdens of decision making in the health service. They respect those who care for them (*see* Box 19.3).

Box 19.3   Characteristics of good citizen–professional interactions

- Manifest consistent technical soundness
- Engage the whole human experience
- Recognise the citizen as a person with unique identity and responsibility
- Use resources appropriately
- Lead to mutually acceptable outcomes
- Help to improve the health of individuals and populations
- Are realistic and affirming
- Share responsibility and decision making

Equally, workers in primary care need to demonstrate their respect for patients, by listening and allowing them the space and the capacity to offer an opinion and to criticise the professional viewpoint as and when appropriate.

Gadamer suggests that, in order to preserve a proper attitude to one's own authority as a professional, one needs to be free to make mistakes on occasions, and to be able to recognise the fact.[20] Appropriate structures of governance must be designed so that they do not inhibit the healer's ability to admit mistakes inwardly, to colleagues or to patients, while at the same time not putting the public at excessive risk. A no-blame, supportive culture with mutuality should be the goal. Without such a culture, governance becomes something to fear, and its presence is seen as an unwarranted imposition. That benefits neither practitioners nor patients.

Practical points

- Idealised definitions of health lead to unrealistic expectations.
- These are fuelled by the pretensions of scientific medicine.
- The challenge for clinical governance is how to improve service quality without encouraging dependency and false expectations among patients.
- Partnership between professionals and citizens points a way forward.
- Patients rightly expect high standards, but also recognise that practitioners are under extreme pressure.
- As citizens they are willing to share decision making with the health service.

References

1   World Health Organization (1948) *The Constitution of the World Health Organization*. World Health Organization, Geneva.
2   Osborne T (1997) Of health and statecraft. In: A Petersen and R Bunton (eds) *Foucault, Health and Medicine*. Routledge, London.
3   World Health Organization and UNICEF (1978) *Primary Health Care (The Alma-Ata Report)*. World Health Organization, Geneva and UNICEF, New York.

4   Seedhouse D (1986) *Health: the foundation for achievement*. John Wiley & Sons, Chichester.

5   Moltmann J (1985) *God in Creation: an ecological doctrine of creation*. SCM Press, London.

6   Campbell AV (1984) *Moderated Love: a theology of professional care*. SPCK, London.

7   Harrison J (1998) Post-modern influences. In: J Harrison and T van Zwanenberg (eds) *GP Tomorrow*. Radcliffe Medical Press, Oxford.

8   Coward R (1999) Go to bed. *The Guardian*. **9 January**.

9   Smith B (1998) *The Silence of Divine Love*. Darton, Longman and Todd, London.

10 Illich I (1995) Death undefeated. From medicine to medicalization to systematization. *BMJ*. **311**: 1652–3.

11 Beck U (1992) *Risk Society: towards a new modernity*. Sage, London.

12 Turner BS (1997) From governmentality to risk. In: A Petersen and R Bunton (eds) *Foucault, Health and Medicine*. Routledge, London.

13 Abelson J, Maxwell PH and Maxwell RJ (1997) Do professions have a future? Perhaps, if they are not defensive or complacent. *BMJ*. **315**: 382.

14 Harrison J (1996) Is this what we really want? *BMJ*. **313**: 1643. *See* also Harrison J and Innes R (1997) *Medical Vocation and Generation X*. Grove Books, Cambridge.

15 Vaughan C and Higgs R (1995) Doctors and commitment. Nice work – shame about the job. *BMJ*. **311**: 1654–5.

16 Jarrold K (1998) *Servants and Leaders: leadership in the NHS*. Lecture, 30 July, University of York, York.

17 Purves I (1998) The changing consultation. In: J Harrison and T van Zwanenberg (eds) *GP Tomorrow*. Radcliffe Medical Press, Oxford.

18 Hermeneutics is the study of interpretation. The hermeneutical process is the task of the doctor or nurse in interpreting the patient's story in the light of both that narrative and the available scientific evidence.

19 Pellegrino ED and Thomasma DC (1981) *A Philosophical Basis of Medical Practice: toward a philosophy and ethic of the healing professions*. Oxford University Press, Oxford.

20 Gadamer H-G (1996) *The Enigma of Health: the art of healing in a scientific age*. Blackwell Science, Oxford.

CHAPTER 20

Implementing clinical governance

Jamie Harrison and Tim van Zwanenberg

For every difficult and complicated question there is an answer that is simple, easily understood and wrong.

HL Mencken

Clinical governance in action

So what, then, is clinical governance? The complementary themes within this book, taken together, seek to paint a picture in which clinical governance is portrayed as the means whereby the issue of quality in primary care can be addressed. Yet each individual and team within primary care may receive the light slanted across the canvas differently, and so perceive the image with slight alterations compared with that of their neighbours.

Or, to take the analogy of the stained glass window, the message of the whole set of panes can change with the quality and quantity of light, the position of the observer and their willingness to engage with the process of looking. Education may be needed in how to interpret the contents of the image, and simplistic answers with regard to what it 'means' will need to be challenged.

For undoubtedly some who claim expertise will appear, offering short-cuts and comfortable options, on the road to clinical governance. Yet common sense dictates that achievement of the proper implementation of clinical governance will take time and effort. Indeed, the Government itself has a 10-year timetable for improving the quality of clinical care.

However, there are decisions to be taken and dilemmas to be resolved in relation to the clinical governance agenda in the here and now. How will primary care begin to measure up to such challenges? And what are the risks it will run should it choose to avoid answering the questions that are being posed?

Communication or confusion?

One significant question for the culture of primary care relates to its willingness to improve communications – both internally and with outsiders. Sadly, patients often fit into the latter grouping. Regular communication within teams, proper consultation mechanisms and effective ways of passing on information lead to a greater ownership of the service by all, more efficiency, less confusion, and (hopefully) better clinical care and job satisfaction.

Humility or hubris?

Both of these words are misunderstood. Humility is misrepresented as weakness; hubris is misrepresented as confident leadership. True humility allows others to make their contribution, values participation in decision making and is willing to learn. Hubris is arrogant power seeking and presumption of unearned authority. The doctor no longer automatically knows what is best for the patient – and the same can be said for any single health professional in primary care.

Courage or complacency?

It is easiest to do nothing, especially in the face of major change. Inertia soon gains the upper hand. There must of course be proper discussion about how to respond to change, with leadership, clarity and time for reflection. The speed of response needs to be measured, with careful planning and realism. However, there may also need to be courage – living out a belief in what is possible, achievable and necessary.

Inclusivity or isolationism?

Should all be included? Does the definition of 'all' need some thought? It is so easy to leave someone out, intentionally or unintentionally. With new primary care team and primary care trust structures in place, work is needed if all are to feel included. Equally, limited horizons can make for delusions of success and false ideas that all is well. We need each other. Strength comes from sharing and seeing the bigger picture, not from being isolated.

Partnership or protectionism?

It is traditional to close ranks when the pressure is on. Professional self-interest is a powerful force, and not only in primary care. Yet the clinical governance agenda calls for the rejection of historical protectionism, replacing it with openness and transparency. Patients, politicians and professionals share many common values and beliefs. Decisions about issues of life and death, the rationing of services and our common future would seem to be more helpfully made together rather than apart.

Conclusion

Clinical governance offers to all in primary care the opportunity to celebrate success as much as to look to improve. It is all too easy to forget that most things are done well, that society values primary care's efforts highly, and that each new generation of doctors, nurses and managers builds on the contribution of its predecessors.

Yet equally there is room to make improvements across the board. Using creativity and simplicity, the new clinical governance agenda can be tackled effectively and systematically. It is, of course, an agenda that is both exciting and not a little daunting.

Index